made INCRED... ...EASY!

Wound Care

Adapted for the UK by
**Julie Vuolo, MA, BA, PG Dip,
Dip PP (TV), RN**

Senior Lecturer,
University of Hertfordshire

First UK Edition

Lippincott Williams & Wilkins

...York • London
...Hong Kong • Sydney • Tokyo

Staff

Director, Global Publishing
Cathy Peck

Production Director
Chris Curtis

Acquisitions Editor
Rachel Hendrick

Project Manager
Cosmas Georgallis

Senior Production Manager
Richard Owen

Academic Marketing Executive
Alison Major

Copy Editor
RTC Editorial

Proofreader
Cosmas Georgallis

Illustrator
Bot Roda

Designer
Designers Collective

Printed and bound by Euradius in The Netherlands. Typeset by Macmillan Publishing Solutions, New Delhi, India

For information, write to Lippincott Williams & Wilkins, 250 Waterloo Road, London SE1 8RD.

British Library Cataloging-in-Publication Data. A catalogue record for this book is available from the British Library.

ISBN13 978-1-901831-06-1
ISBN10 1-901831-06-X

Contents

Acknowledgements

Contributors

Irene Anderson, MSc, BSc(Hons), DPSN, PGCE, RN, LPE, FHEA
Senior Lecturer, University of Hertfordshire,
Hatfield, Hertfordshire, UK
Adapted chapter 10, 'Leg Ulcers'

Jacqui Fletcher, MSc, BSc(Hons), PGCE, RN, FHEA
Principal Lecturer, University of Hertfordshire,
Hatfield, Hertfordshire, UK
Adapted chapter 8, 'Pressure Ulcers'

Jane Leaver, BSc(Hons), RN
Lecturer Practitioner, Birmingham City University
Provided guidance on plastics and burns

Reviewers of the UK edition

Iwan Dowie, BSc, Dip HE, LLB, PgD, PGCE, RN
Senior Lecturer, University of Glamorgan, Wales

Jane James, MSc, Dip DN, PGCE, RN
Tissue Viability Nurse, Hywell Dda Nhs Trust, Wales

Zena Moore, MSc, RN, FFNM (RCSI)
Research Fellow, Royal College of Surgeons in Ireland

Foreword

Wound care is a dynamic, constantly changing field that crosses all specialties and age groups. In recent years, interest in the field has grown substantially and now many different healthcare professions, including nursing, medicine, physiotherapy and dietetics are working together to improve patient outcomes. Recognition that acute and non-healing wounds greatly impact on quality of life as well as financial aspects of our healthcare system has raised the profile of wound care and led to the development of many special interest groups. In the UK and beyond, healthcare professionals are now working hard to ensure high quality care is available to all patients who have or are at risk of having a wound.

Wound Care Made Incredibly Easy!, First UK Edition, is an impressive reference for both the beginner and experienced practitioner. Theoretical as well as practical aspects of wound management are addressed within the text. A review of basic skin anatomy and physiology provides a foundation for understanding various acute and non-healing wound aetiologies. Chapters discussing treatment and dressing methodologies build on this knowledge and allow the practitioner to employ evidence-based wound care. This edition has been substantially revised throughout and includes a new chapter on accountability and legal issues and chapter by chapter key references.

On top of that, it's fun! Illustrations, photographs and charts present need-to-know concepts and procedures in an easy-to-understand and easy-to-read format. Two sections of colour pages bring you a dramatic view of common wound types and complications as well as guiding you through pressure ulcer categorisation. Appendices, such as the quick guide to wound care dressings and the wound and skin assessment tool, serve as tools you can use in your practice again and again. Quick quizzes at the end of each chapter test your knowledge and lighthearted characters throughout the book make learning fun and enjoyable.

Entertaining logos highlight key points:

Dress for success presents tips for choosing and applying wound dressings.

Get wise to wounds provides pointers for performing wound assessment, wound care procedures and patient teaching.

Handle with care explains the unique wound care needs of vulnerable patient groups.

Memory joggers offer mnemonic devices and other learning aids to help reinforce difficult topics.

A quality wound management reference must address the needs of the wide variety of professionals in wound care. *Wound Care Made Incredibly Easy!*, First UK Edition, is a well-thought-out reference that provides sound information to benefit the expert and novice alike.

Julie Vuolo, MA, BA, PG Dip, Dip PP (TV), RN
Senior Lecturer
Tissue Viability
University of Hertfordshire
Hatfield, UK

Contributors and consultants to the US edition

Monica A. Beshara, RN, BSN, CWOCN
Wound Care Specialist
DeKalb Medical Center
Decatur, Ga.

Phyllis A. Bonham, PhD, RN, MSN, CWOCN
Associate Professor and Director, Wound Care Education Program
College of Nursing
Medical University of South Carolina
Charleston

Carol Calianno, RN, MSN, CWOCN
Wound, Ostomy, Continence Nurse Specialist
Jeanes Hospital — Temple Health System
Philadelphia

Margaret Davis, RN, MSN, PhD(c)
Assistant Professor of Nursing
Central Florida Community College
Ocala

Roxanne Leisky, MSN, MBA, FNP, CWS
Owner
Advanced Wound Care, LLC
Springfield, Ill.

Donna Scemons, RN, MSN, FNP-C, CWOCN, CNS
Family Nurse Practitioner
Healthcare Systems Inc.
Castaic, Calif.

Tracey J. Siegel, RN, MSN, CWOCN, NP
Instructor of Nursing
Charles E. Gregory School of Nursing
Perth Amboy, N.J.

Mary Sieggreen, APRN-BC, MSN, CVN
Nurse Practitioner Vascular Surgery
Harper University Hospital, Detroit Medical Center

Patricia Albano Slachta, APRN, BC, PHD, CWOCN
Clinical Nurse Specialist
Medical University of South Carolina
Charleston

Cynthia A. Worley, RN, BSN, COCN, CWCN
WOC Nurse
University of Texas M.D. Anderson Cancer Center
Houston

Karen Zulkowski, RN, DNS, CWS
Associate Professor
Montana State University
Bozeman

1 Wound care fundamentals

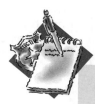

Just the facts

In this chapter, you'll learn:
- layers and functions of the skin
- types of wounds
- phases of wound healing
- factors that affect the skin's ability to heal
- complications of wound healing.

A look at the skin

The skin, or integumentary system, is the largest organ in the body. It accounts for about 6 to 8 lb (2.5 to 3.5 kg) of a person's body weight and has a surface area of more than 20 square feet. The thickest skin is located on the hands and on the soles of the feet; the thinnest skin, around the eyes and over the tympanic membranes in the ears.

Beauty's only skin deep

Skin protects the body by acting as a barrier between internal structures and the external world. Because skin also stands between each of us and the social world around us, we're also affected by its appearance. Healthy, unblemished skin with good tone (firmness) and colour leads to a better self image. Skin also reflects the body's general physical health. For example, skin may look bluish if blood oxygen levels are low and it may appear flushed or red if a fever is present.

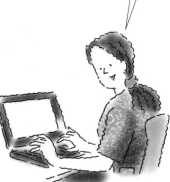

Wow! The skin makes up 6 to 8 lb of a person's weight. That's more than this laptop weighs!

A wound by any other name

Any break in the continuity of the skin is considered a wound. Wounds to the skin can result from planned events (such as surgery), accidents (such as a fall from a bike) or exposure to the environment (such as the damage caused by ultraviolet (UV) rays in sunlight).

Anatomy and physiology

Skin is composed of two main layers that function as a single unit: the epidermis and the dermis. The epidermis (outermost layer) is made up of five distinct layers. Covering the epidermis is the keratinised epithelium, a layer of cells that migrate up from the underlying dermis and die upon reaching the surface. These cells are continuously generated and replaced. The dermis (innermost layer) is made up of living cells that receive oxygen and nutrients through an extensive network of small blood vessels. In fact, every square inch of skin contains more than 4.5 metres of blood vessels! A layer of subcutaneous fatty connective tissue, sometimes called the hypodermis, lies beneath these layers.

When my melanin kicks in, I'll be sporting a nice tan, but maybe I should start sporting some sunblock. These UV rays can be pretty damaging.

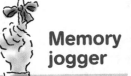

The skin you're in

Within the epidermis and dermis are five structural networks:
- collagen fibres
- elastic fibres
- small blood vessels
- nerve fibres
- lymphatic vessels.

These networks are stabilised by hair follicles and sweat gland ducts.

Epidermis

The epidermis – the outermost of the skin's two main layers – varies in thickness from about 0.1 mm thick on the eyelids to as much as 1 mm thick on the palms and soles. It's slightly acidic, with an average pH of 5.5.

In living colour

The epidermis also contains melanocytes (cells that produce the brown pigment melanin), which give skin and hair their colours. The more melanin produced by melanocytes, the darker the skin. Skin colour varies from one person to the next, but it can also vary from one area of the body to another. The hypothalamus regulates melanin production by secreting melanocyte-stimulating hormone.

Memory jogger

Keep the skin layers straight by remembering that the prefix **epi-** means 'upon'. Therefore, the epidermis is upon, or on top of, the dermis.

The layered look

Each of the five layers of the epidermis has a name that reflects either its structure or its function. Let's look at them from the outside in:

• The *stratum corneum* (horny layer) is the superficial layer of dead skin cells (keratinised epithelium) that's in contact with the environment. This layer is separated by the dermis and underlying tissue. The stratum corneum has an acid mantle that helps protect the body from some fungi and bacteria. Cells in this layer continuously migrate through the stratum lucidum from the dermis below and die upon reaching the surface. These dead cells are shed daily and are completely replaced every 4 to 6 weeks. In diseases, such as eczema and psoriasis, the stratum corneum may become abnormally thick and irritate skin structures and peripheral nerves.

• The *stratum lucidum* (clear layer) is a single layer of cells that forms a transitional boundary between the stratum corneum above and stratum granulosum below. This layer is most evident in areas where skin is thickest such as on the soles. It appears to be absent in areas where skin is especially thin such as on the eyelids. Although cells in this layer lack active nuclei, this is an area of intense enzyme activity that prepares cells for the stratum corneum.

• The *stratum granulosum* (granular layer) is one to five cells thick and is characterised by flat cells with active nuclei. It's believed that this layer aids keratin formation.

• The *stratum spinosum* is the layer in which cells begin to flatten as they migrate towards the skin surface. Involucrin, a soluble protein precursor of the keratinised envelopes of skin cells, is synthesised here.

• The *stratum basale*, or *stratum germinativum*, is just one cell thick and is the only layer of the epidermis in which cells undergo mitosis to form new cells. The stratum basale forms the dermoepidermal junction – the area where the epidermis and dermis are connected. Protrusions of this layer (called *rete pegs* or *epidermal ridges*) extend down into the dermis where they're surrounded by vascularised dermal papillae. This unique structure supports the epidermis and facilitates the exchange of fluids and cells between the skin layers.

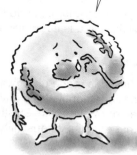

It's time for me to migrate to the skin's surface. I'll miss you stratum spinosum!

Dermis

The dermis – the thick, deeper layer of the skin – is composed of collagen and elastin fibres and an extracellular matrix, which contributes to the skin's strength and pliability. Collagen fibres give skin its strength, and elastin fibres provide elasticity. The meshing of collagen and elastin determines the skin's physical characteristics. (See *Structural supports: collagen and elastin*.)

In addition, the dermis contains:

- blood vessels and lymphatic vessels, which transport oxygen and nutrients to cells and remove waste products
- nerve fibres and hair follicles, which contribute to skin sensation, temperature regulation and excretion and absorption through the skin
- fibroblast cells, which are important in the production of collagen and elastin.

Structural supports: collagen and elastin

After you pull on the skin, it normally returns to its original position. This is because of the actions of the connective tissues collagen and elastin – two key components of skin.

Understanding the components

Collagen and elastin work together to support the dermis and give skin its physical characteristics.

Collagen

Collagen fibres form tightly woven networks in the papillary layer of the dermis – thick bundles that run parallel to the skin's surface. These fibres are relatively inextensible and nonelastic; therefore, they give the dermis high tensile strength. In addition, collagen constitutes about 70% of the skin's dry weight and is its principal structural body protein.

Elastin

Elastin is made up of wavy fibres that intertwine with collagen in horizontal arrangements at the lower dermis and vertical arrangements at the epidermal margin. Elastin makes skin pliable and is the structural protein that enables extensibility in the dermis.

Seeing the effects of age

As a person ages, collagen and elastin fibres break down and the fine lines and wrinkles that are associated with ageing develop. Extensive exposure to sunlight accelerates this breakdown process. Deep wrinkles are caused by changes in facial muscles. Over time, laughing, crying, smiling and frowning cause facial muscles to thicken and eventually cause wrinkles in the overlying skin.

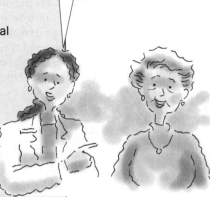

Don't let your laugh lines give you worry warts. Breakdown of collagen and elastin fibres is a normal part of ageing.

It takes two

The dermis is composed of two layers of connective tissue:
- The *papillary dermis* (outermost layer) is composed of collagen and reticular fibres, which are important in healing wounds. Capillaries in the papillary dermis carry the nourishment needed for metabolic activity in this layer.
- The *reticular dermis* (innermost layer) is formed by thick networks of collagen bundles that anchor it to the subcutaneous tissue and underlying supporting structures (such as fasciae, muscle and bone).

Sebaceous glands and sweat glands

Although sebaceous glands and sweat glands appear to originate in the dermis, they're actually appendages of the epidermis that extend downwards into the dermis.

Give these glands a hand!

Sebaceous glands, found primarily in the skin of the scalp, face, upper body and genital region, are part of the same structure that contains hair follicles. These sac-like glands produce sebum, a fatty substance that lubricates and softens the skin.

Don't sweat it

Sweat glands are tightly coiled and tubular; the average person has roughly 2.6 million of them. They're present throughout the body in varying amounts: the palms and soles have many but the external ear, lip margins, nail beds and glans penis have none.

The secreting portion of the sweat gland originates in the dermis with its outlet on the surface of the skin. The sympathetic nervous system regulates sweat production, which, in turn, helps control body temperature.

Two types of sweat glands are present:
- *Eccrine* glands are active at birth and are found throughout the body. They're most dense on the palms, soles and forehead. These glands connect to the skin's surface through pores and produce sweat that lacks proteins and fatty acids. Eccrine glands are smaller than apocrine glands.
- *Apocrine* glands begin to function at puberty. These glands open into hair follicles; therefore, most are found in areas where hair typically grows, such as the scalp, groin and axillary region. The coiled secreting portion of each gland lies deep in the dermis (deeper than eccrine glands), and a duct connects it to the upper portion of the hair follicle. The sweat produced by apocrine glands contains water, sodium, chloride, proteins and fatty acids. It's thicker than the sweat produced by eccrine glands and has a milky-white or yellowish tinge. (See *Oh no, B.O.!* page 6.)

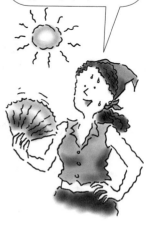

Along with this fan, my sympathetic nervous system helps keep me cool on hot days like this one. It really is 'sympathetic', isn't it?

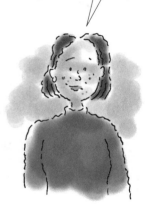

Apocrine sweat glands begin to function at puberty. Lucky me!

Oh no, B.O.!

The sweat produced by apocrine glands contains the same water, sodium and chloride found in the sweat produced by eccrine glands; however, it also contains proteins and fatty acids. The unpleasant odour associated with sweat comes from the interaction of bacteria with these proteins and fatty acids.

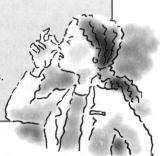

Subcutaneous tissue

Subcutaneous tissue, or hypodermis, is the subdermal (below the skin) layer of loose connective tissue that contains major blood vessels, lymph vessels and nerves. Subcutaneous tissue:
* has a high proportion of fat cells and contains fewer small blood vessels than the dermis
* varies in thickness depending on body type and location
* constitutes 15% to 20% of a man's weight; 20% to 25% of a woman's weight
* insulates the body
* absorbs shocks to the skeletal system
* helps skin move easily over underlying structures.

Blood supply

The skin receives its blood supply through vessels that originate in underlying muscle tissue. Here, arteries branch into smaller vessels, which then branch into the network of capillaries that permeate the dermis and subcutaneous tissue.

Just passing through

Within the vascular system, only capillaries have walls thin enough (typically only a single layer of endothelial cells) to let solutes pass through. These thin walls allow nutrients and oxygen to pass from the bloodstream into the interstitial space around skin cells. At the same time, waste products pass into the capillaries and are carried away. The pressure of arterial blood entering the capillaries is about 30 mmHg. The pressure of venous blood leaving the capillaries is about 10 mmHg. This 20 mmHg difference in pressure within the capillaries is quite low when compared with the pressure found in the larger arteries in the body (85 to 100 mmHg), which is known as *blood pressure*. (See *Fluid movement through capillaries*, page 7.)

Fluid movement through capillaries

The movement of fluids through capillaries – a process called capillary filtration – results from blood pushing against the walls of the capillary. That pressure, called hydrostatic or fluid-pushing pressure, forces fluids and solutes through the capillary wall.

When the hydrostatic pressure inside a capillary is greater than the pressure in the surrounding interstitial space, fluids and solutes inside the capillary are forced out into the interstitial space, as shown here. When the pressure inside the capillary is less than the pressure outside, fluids and solutes move back into it.

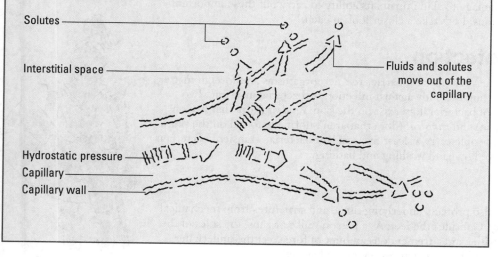

Solutes

Interstitial space

Fluids and solutes
move out of the
capillary

Hydrostatic pressure

Capillary

Capillary wall

Lymphatic system

The skin's lymphatic system helps remove waste products, including excess proteins and fluids, from the dermis.

Go with the flow

Lymphatic vessels, or *lymphatics* for short, are similar to capillaries in that they're thin-walled, permeable vessels; however, lymphatics aren't part of the blood circulatory system. Instead, lymphatics belong to a separate system that removes proteins, large waste products and excess fluids from the interstitial spaces in skin and then transports them to the venous circulation. The lymphatic vessels merge into two main trunks – the thoracic duct and the right lymphatic duct – which empty into the junction of the subclavian and internal jugular veins.

Functions of the skin

Skin performs, or participates in, a host of vital functions, including:
- protection of internal structures
- sensory perception
- thermoregulation
- excretion
- metabolism
- absorption
- social communication.

Damage to skin impairs its ability to carry out these important functions. Let's take a closer look at each.

Protection

Skin acts as a physical barrier to microorganisms and foreign matter, protecting the body against infection by bacterial invasion. Two kinds of bacterial flora exist on the skin: *resident* (flora that live on the skin) and *transient* (flora that aren't normally found on the skin). Most people carry at least five resident bacteria. Transient bacteria is removed by hand washing and bathing.

A thick skin

Skin also protects underlying tissue and structures from mechanical injury. Consider the feet: As a person walks or runs, the soles of the feet withstand a tremendous amount of force, yet the underlying tissue and bone structures remain unharmed.

Sensational stability

Finally, skin helps maintain a stable environment inside the body by preventing the loss of water, electrolytes, proteins and other substances. Any damage jeopardises this protection. When it's damaged, skin goes into repair mode to restore full protection by stepping up the normal process of cell replacement.

Sensory perception

Nerve endings in the skin allow a person to literally feel the world around them. Sensory nerve fibres originate in the nerve roots along the spine and supply specific areas of the skin known as *dermatomes*. Dermatomes are used to transmit sensory function. This same network helps a person avoid injury by making them aware of pain, pressure, heat and cold.

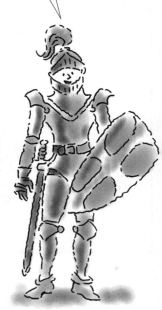

Sometimes you need more protection than at other times. Skin acts as a physical barrier to such invaders as microorganisms.

Sensitivity training

Sensory nerves exist throughout the skin; however, some areas are more sensitive than others – for example, the fingertips are more sensitive than the back. Sensation allows us to identify potential dangers and avoid injury. Any loss or reduction of sensation (local or general) increases the chance of injury.

Thermoregulation

Thermoregulation, or control of body temperature, involves the concerted effort of nerves, blood vessels and eccrine glands in the dermis. When skin is exposed to cold or internal body temperature falls, blood vessels constrict, reducing blood flow and thereby conserving body heat. Similarly, if skin becomes too hot or internal body temperature rises, small arteries within the skin dilate, increasing the blood flow, and sweat production increases to promote cooling.

Excretion

Although it may seem unlikely, the skin is an excretory organ. Excretion through the skin plays an important role in thermoregulation, electrolyte balance and hydration. In addition, sebum excretion helps maintain the skin's integrity and suppleness.

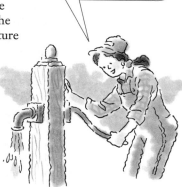

Sweat carries water to the skin's surface, at the same time preventing dehydration by making sure the body doesn't lose too much water.

Water works

Through its more than two million pores (small openings in the skin where sebum and sweat are released), the skin efficiently transmits trace amounts of water and body wastes to the environment. At the same time, it prevents dehydration by ensuring that the body doesn't lose too much water. Sweat carries water and salt to the skin surface, where it evaporates, aiding thermoregulation and electrolyte balance. In addition, a small amount of water evaporates directly from the skin itself each day. A normal adult loses about 500 ml of water a day this way. While the skin is busy regulating fluids that are leaving the body through sweat production, it's equally busy preventing unwanted or dangerous fluids from entering the body.

Metabolism

Skin also helps to maintain the mineralisation of bones and teeth.

A photochemical reaction in the skin produces vitamin D, which is crucial to the metabolism of calcium and phosphate. These minerals, in turn, play a central role in the health of bones and teeth. When skin is exposed to the UV spectrum in sunlight, vitamin D is synthesised in a photochemical reaction. Keep in mind, however, that overexposure to UV light causes damage that reduces the skin's ability to function properly.

Absorption

Some drugs and toxic substances (for example, pesticides) can be absorbed directly through the skin and into the bloodstream. This absorption process has been used to treat certain disorders via skin patch drug delivery systems. One example is the transdermal drug delivery method used in some nicotine withdrawal programs. This technology is also used to administer some forms of contraception, hormone replacement therapy, nitroglycerin and some pain medications.

Social communication

A commonly overlooked but important function of the skin is its role in self-esteem development and social communication. Every time a person looks in the mirror, he decides whether he likes what he sees. Although bone structure, body type, teeth and hair all have an impact, the condition and characteristics of the skin can have the greatest impact on a person's self-esteem. Ask any teenager with acne. If a person likes what he sees, self-esteem rises; if he doesn't, it sags.

You should have seen your face

Virtually every interpersonal exchange includes the nonverbal languages of facial expression and body posture. A person's level of self-esteem and skin characteristics – which are visible at all times – have an impact on how he communicates, both verbally and nonverbally, and how he's received by a listener. Because the physical characteristics of skin are so closely linked to self-perception, a proliferation of skin care products and surgical techniques are available to keep skin looking young and healthy.

Ageing and skin function

Over time, skin loses its ability to function as efficiently or as effectively as it once did. (See *How skin ages*, page 11.) As a result, advanced age places a person at greater risk of skin injury, such as pressure ulcers and skin tears, and increases the risks of delayed healing.

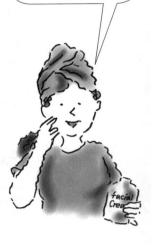

I'm not sure how I look right now, but I'm on my way to younger and healthier looking skin, according to the bottle. Watch out world!

Handle with care

How skin ages

This table lists skin changes that normally occur with ageing.

Change	Findings in elderly patients
Pigmentation	• Pale colour
Thickness	• Wrinkling, especially on the face, arms and legs • Parchment-like appearance, especially over bony prominences and on the dorsal surfaces of the hands, feet, arms and legs
Moisture	• Dry, flaky and rough
Turgor	• 'Tents' and stands alone
Texture	• Numerous creases and lines

As a person ages, skin undergoes many changes that can increase the risk of wounds.

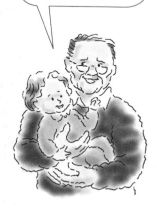

The road ahead

Although the entire body changes a great deal over time, several important changes in the skin increase the risk of wounds as a person ages. These include:
• a 50% reduction in the cell turnover rate in the stratum corneum (outermost layer) and a 20% reduction in dermal thickness
• generalised reduction in dermal vascularisation and an associated drop in blood flow to the skin
• redistribution of subcutaneous tissue, which contains fewer fat cells in older people, to the stomach and thighs
• flattening of papillae in the dermoepidermal junction (meeting of the epidermis and dermis), which reduces adhesion between layers
• a drop in the number of Langerhans' cells (cells that attack invading germs) present in the skin
• a 50% decline in the number of fibroblasts and mast cells (cells that play a key role in the inflammatory response)
• marked reduction in the ability to sense pressure, heat and cold, even though the same number of nerve endings in the skin are retained
• a significant decline in the number of sweat glands
• poorer absorption through the skin
• a reduction in the skin's ability to synthesise vitamin D.

Injury alert

As a person ages, physiological changes also increase the risk of various skin-related injuries. For example, older adults:
- bruise more easily and are more prone to oedema around wounds due to reduced skin vascularisation
- are more likely to suffer pressure and thermal (hot and cold) damage to the skin due to diminished sensation
- have a higher incidence of ischaemia (cell damage resulting from too little oxygen reaching cells) in compressed tissue because bony areas have less subcutaneous cushioning and decreased sensation causes an elderly person to be less sensitive to the discomfort of remaining in one position for too long
- risk hyperthermia and hypothermia because of decreased subcutaneous tissue
- have fewer sweat glands and, therefore, produce less sweat, which hinders thermoregulation and increases the risk of hyperthermia
- have a higher risk of infection because thinner skin is a less effective barrier to germs and allergens and because the skin contains fewer Langerhans' cells to fight infection and fewer mast cells to mediate the inflammatory response
- are slower to exhibit a sensitisation response (redness, heat, discomfort) due to the reduction in Langerhans' cells, resulting in overuse of topical medications and more severe allergic reactions (because signs aren't evident early on)
- risk overdose of transdermal medications when poor absorption prompts them to reapply the medication too often
- have a much higher incidence of shear and tear injuries due to compromised skin layer adhesion and less flexible collagen.

A look at wounds

Any break in the skin is considered a wound. Tissue damage in wounds varies widely, from a superficial break in the epithelium to deep trauma that involves the muscle and bone. A 'clean' wound is a wound produced by surgery. A wound is described as 'dirty' if it contains bacteria or other debris. Traumatic injury typically produces dirty wounds. The rate of wound recovery varies according to the extent and type of damage incurred and intrinsic factors such as the patient's circulation, nutrition and hydration. Although the recovery rate varies, the healing process is much the same in all cases.

Trauma can cause some pretty dirty wounds.

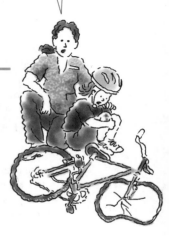

Types of wound healing

A wound may be classified by the way it closes. A wound can be closed by primary, secondary or tertiary intention.

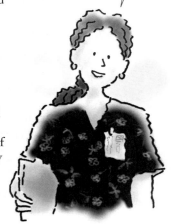

Wounds may heal by primary, secondary or tertiary intention.

Primary intention

Primary intention involves re-epithelialisation, in which the skin's outer layer closes over the wound. Cells grow in from the margins of the wound and out from epithelial cells lining the hair follicles and sweat glands.

Just a scratch

Wounds that heal by primary intention are, most commonly, superficial wounds that involve only the epidermis with no loss of dermal tissue – a superficial (first degree) burn for example. A wound that has well-approximated edges (edges that can be pulled together to meet neatly), such as a surgical incision, also heals by primary intention. Because there's no loss of tissue and little risk of infection, the healing process is predictable. These wounds usually heal in 4 to 21 days and result in minimal scarring.

Secondary intention

Wounds that involve some degree of tissue loss with edges that can't be easily approximated heal by secondary intention. Depending on a wound's depth, it can be described as partial thickness or full thickness:
• Partial-thickness wounds extend through the epidermis and into, but not through, the dermis.
• Full-thickness wounds extend through the epidermis and dermis and may involve subcutaneous tissue, muscle and, possibly, bone.

Skin deep

During healing, wounds that heal by secondary intention fill with granulation tissue; then re-epithelialisation occurs, primarily from the wound edges, and finally a scar forms. Pressure ulcers, burns, dehisced surgical wounds and traumatic injuries are examples of this type of wound. These wounds take longer to heal, result in scarring, and have a higher rate of complications than wounds that heal by primary intention.

Tertiary intention

Wounds that are intentionally kept open to allow oedema or infection to resolve or to permit removal of exudate heal by tertiary intention (also called *delayed primary intention*). These wounds are later closed with sutures, staples or adhesive skin closures. Wounds that heal by tertiary intention often result in more scarring than wounds that heal by primary intention but less than wounds that heal by secondary intention.

Phases of wound healing

Whether the cause is mechanical, chemical or thermal, the healing process is the same for all wounds. The wound healing process involves four specific phases:
- haemostasis
- inflammation
- proliferation
- maturation.

Although this categorisation is useful, it's important to remember that typically, the phases of wound healing overlap. (See *How wounds heal*, page 15.)

Haemostasis

Immediately after an injury, the body releases chemical mediators and intercellular messengers called *growth factors* that begin the process of cleaning and healing the wound.

Slow that flow!

When blood vessels are damaged, the small muscles in the walls of the vessels contract (vasoconstriction), reducing the flow of blood to the injury and minimising blood loss. The arrest of bleeding by vasoconstriction is known as *haemostasis*. Vasoconstriction can last as long as 30 minutes.

Next, blood leaking from the inflamed, dilated or broken vessels begins to coagulate. Collagen fibres in the wall of the damaged blood vessels activate the platelets in the blood that's in the wound. Aided by the action of prostaglandins, the platelets enlarge and stick together to form a temporary plug in the blood vessel, which helps prevent further bleeding. The platelets also release additional vasoconstrictors, such as serotonin, which help to prevent further blood loss. Thrombin forms in a cascade of events stimulated by the platelets, and a clot forms to close the small vessels and stop bleeding.

The initial phase of wound healing occurs almost immediately after the injury occurs and works quickly (within minutes) in small wounds. Haemostasis is less effective in stopping the bleeding in larger wounds.

Vasoconstriction reduces the flow of blood to the injury, minimising blood loss and promoting haemostasis.

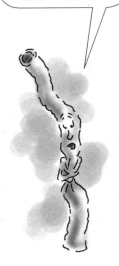

How wounds heal

The healing process begins at the instant of injury and proceeds through a repair 'cascade', as outlined here.

1. When tissue is damaged, serotonin, histamine, prostaglandins and blood from the injured vessels fill the area. Blood platelets form a clot, and fibrin in the clot binds the wound edges together.

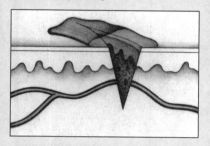

2. Lymphocytes initiate the inflammatory response, increasing capillary permeability. Wound edges swell; white blood cells from surrounding vessels move in and ingest bacteria and cellular debris, demolishing the clot. Redness, warmth, swelling, pain and loss of function may occur.

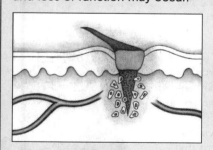

3. Adjacent healthy tissue supplies blood, nutrients, fibroblasts, proteins and other building materials needed to form soft, pink and highly vascular granulation tissue, which begins to bridge the area. Inflammation may decrease, or signs and symptoms of infection (increased swelling, increased pain, fever and pus-filled discharge) may develop.

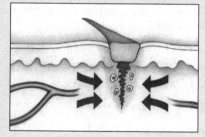

4. Fibroblasts in the granulation tissue secrete collagen, a glue-like substance. Collagen fibres criss-cross the area, forming scar tissue.

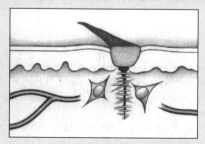

Meanwhile, epithelial cells at the wound edge multiply and migrate towards the wound centre. A new layer of surface cells replaces the layer that was destroyed. New, healthy tissue or granulation tissue (if the blood supply is inadequate) appears.

5. Damaged tissue (including lymphatics, blood vessels, and stromal matrices) regenerates. Collagen fibres shorten, and the scar diminishes in size. Scar size may decrease and normal function may return or the scar may hypertrophy, leading to the formation of a keloid and the development of contractures.

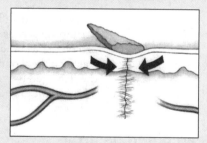

Inflammation

The inflammatory phase is both a defence mechanism and a crucial component of the healing process in which the wound is cleaned and rebuilding begins. (See *Understanding the inflammatory response*, page 16.)

Understanding the inflammatory response

This flowchart outlines the sequence of events in the inflammatory process.

Microorganisms invade damaged tissue.

Basophils release heparin, and histamine and kinin production occurs.

Vasodilation occurs along with increased capillary permeability.

Blood flow increases to the affected tissues and fluid collects within them.

Neutrophils flock to the invasion site to engulf and destroy microorganisms from dying cells.

This sets the stage for the next phase: proliferation.

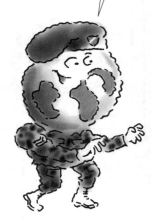

My mission's code name is phagocytosis. My orders are to infiltrate wounds and remove and destroy contaminants.

During the inflammatory phase, vascular permeability increases, permitting serous fluid carrying small amounts of cell and plasma protein to accumulate in the tissue around the wound (oedema) and leak into the wound bed (exudate). The accumulation of fluid causes the damaged tissue to appear swollen, red and warm to the touch. The patient may complain of discomfort or pain around the site of injury.

Search and destroy

During the early phase of the inflammatory process, neutrophils (one type of white blood cell) enter the wound. The primary role of neutrophils is phagocytosis (removal and destruction of bacteria and other contaminants).

As neutrophil infiltration slows, monocytes, another type of white blood cell, appear. Monocytes are converted into activated macrophages and continue the job of cleaning the wound. The macrophages also play a key role early in the process of granulation and re-epithelialisation by producing growth factors and by attracting the cells needed for the formation of new blood vessels and collagen.

Telling time

The inflammatory phase of healing is important for preventing wound infection. The process is negatively influenced if the patient has a systemic condition that suppresses their immune system or if they are undergoing immunosuppressive therapy. In clean wounds, the inflammatory response lasts about 36 hours. In dirty or infected wounds, the response can last much longer.

Proliferation

During the proliferation phase of the healing process, the body:
- fills the wound with connective tissue (granulation)
- contracts the wound edges (contraction)
- covers the wound with epithelium (epithelialisation).

All change!

All wounds go through the proliferation phase, but it takes much longer in wounds with extensive tissue loss. Although phases overlap, wound granulation generally starts when the inflammatory response is complete. As the inflammatory phase subsides, wound exudate (drainage), pain and oedema begin to decrease.

The proliferation phase involves regeneration of blood vessels (angiogenesis) and the formation of connective or granulation tissue. The development of granulation tissue requires an adequate supply of blood and nutrients. Endothelial cells in the blood vessels of the surrounding tissue reconstruct damaged or destroyed vessels by first migrating and then proliferating to form new capillary beds. As the beds form, this area of the wound takes on a red, 'beefy', granular appearance. This tissue is a good defence against contaminants, but it's also quite fragile and bleeds easily.

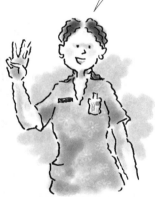

Granulation, contraction and epithelialisation are the three stages of the proliferation phase.

Let the rebuilding begin

During the proliferation phase, growth factors prompt fibroblasts to migrate to the wound. Fibroblasts are the most common cell in connective tissue. They're responsible for making new fibres and ground substance (also known as *extracellular matrix*), which provides support to cells. At first, fibroblasts populate just the margins of the wound; they later spread over the entire wound surface.

Fibroblasts have the important task of synthesising collagen fibres which, in turn, produce keratinocyte, a growth factor needed for re-epithelialisation. This process necessitates a delicate balance of collagen synthesis and lysis (making new and removing old collagen). If the process yields too much collagen, increased scarring results. If the process yields too little collagen, scar tissue is weak and easily ruptured. Because fibroblasts require a supply of oxygen to perform their important role, capillary bed regeneration is crucial to the process.

Pulling it all together

As healing progresses, myofibroblasts and the newly formed collagen fibres contract, pulling the wound edges towards each other. Contraction reduces the amount of granulation tissue needed to fill the wound, which speeds the healing process. (See *Contraction vs. contracture.*)

Complete healing occurs only after epithelial cells have completely covered the surface of the wound. When this occurs, keratinocytes switch from a migratory mode to a differentiation mode. The epidermis thickens and becomes differentiated and the wound is closed. Any remaining scab comes off and the new epidermis is toughened by the production of keratin, which also returns the skin to its original colour.

Maturation

The final phase of wound healing is maturation, which is marked externally by the shrinking and strengthening of the scar and internally by the remodelling (strengthening) and reorganisation of the collagen fibres which make up the new skin tissue.

> Fibroblasts may be small but we have a big job. We synthesise collagen, which is necessary for proper wound healing.

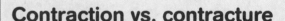

Contraction vs. contracture

Contraction and contracture occur during the wound healing process. While they have mechanisms in common, it's important to understand how contraction and contracture differ:

- *Contraction* is a desirable process that occurs during healing, is the process by which the edges of a wound pull toward the centre of the wound to close it. Contraction continues to close the wound until tension in the surrounding skin causes it to slow and then stop.
- *Contracture* is an undesirable process and a common complication of burn scarring. Typically, contracture occurs after healing is complete. Contracture involves an inordinate amount of pulling or shortening of tissue, resulting in an area of tissue with only limited ability to move. It's especially problematic over joints, which may be pulled to a flexed position. Stretching is the only way to overcome contracture, and patients typically require physical therapy.

Moving on

During maturation, fibroblasts leave the site of the wound, vascularisation is reduced, the scar shrinks and becomes pale and the mature scar forms. If the wound involved extensive tissue destruction, the scar won't contain hair, sweat or sebaceous glands.

The wound gradually gains in tensile strength although it never returns fully to its pre-injury status, even in the healthiest of patients (Forester *et al.* 1969). Scar tissue will always be less elastic than the surrounding skin affecting not only tensile strength but also the appearance and function of the injured site. Some patients are further affected by advanced age and poor nutritional status. The tensile strength of wounds in patients in the sixth decade of life and beyond and those with low serum albumin levels have been reported as significantly lower than would otherwise be expected (Lindstedt and Sandblom 1975).

Maturation is a gradual, transitional phase of healing that can continue for months or even years after the wound has closed. It is important that your patient understands this and knows that symptoms such as itching and tingling, due to collagen fibre remodelling and reorganisation, are both common and normal.

Patients should be made aware of how to seek professional advice if they are concerned about any stage of the healing process including the late stages of maturation which may continue long after the patient has been discharged.

Factors that affect healing

The healing process is affected by many factors. The most important influences include:

- nutrition
- oxygenation
- infection
- age
- chronic health conditions
- medications
- smoking
- socioeconomic factors
- psychological factors.

Nutrition

Proper nutrition is one of the most important factors in successful, uncomplicated wound healing. Poor nutrition or specifically malnutrition will impact on healing in a variety of ways. Malnutrition is a state which normally refers to a deficiency of nutrients such as energy, protein, vitamins and minerals which causes measurable adverse effects on body composition, function or clinical outcome (NICE 2006).

Malnutrition is a common finding among older adults and hospitalised patients. A national survey of community dwelling adults over the age of 65 showed 10% ate inadequate energy-giving foods, whilst 15% of residential home patients were underweight (Martin 2001). The prevalence of malnutrition on admission to hospital has been reported as being between 20% and 40% (Potter *et al.* 1995) and as between 13% and 78% for acute in-patients (Holmes 2007).

Poor nutrition prolongs hospitalisation and increases the risk of medical complications. The severity of complications is directly related to the severity of the malnutrition. In older patients, malnutrition is known to increase the risk of pressure ulcers and delay wound healing. It may also contribute to poor tensile strength in healing wounds, with an associated increase in the risk of wound dehiscence (Lindstedt and Sandblom 1975). (See *Tips for detecting nutritional problems*, page 21.)

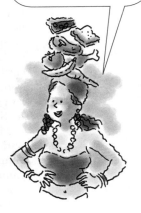

Because nutrition plays a critical role in wound healing, you need to make sure that your patient eats a balanced diet.

Protein power

Protein is crucial for wounds to heal properly. In fact, a person needs to double the recommended dietary allowance of protein (from 0.8 to 1.6 g/kg/day) before tissue even begins to heal. If a significant amount of body weight has been lost in connection with the injury, as much as 50% of the lost weight must be regained before healing will begin. A patient who lacks protein reserves heals slowly, if at all, and a patient who's borderline malnourished can easily become malnourished under this demand.

The body needs protein to form collagen during the proliferation phase. Without adequate protein, collagen formation is reduced or delayed and the healing process slows. Studies of malnourished patients indicate that they have lower levels of serum albumin, which results in slower oxygen diffusion and, in turn, a reduction in the ability of neutrophils to kill bacteria. Chronic wound exudate, in particular, usually contains high levels of protein and this, in turn, can contribute to decreased albumin levels.

Nifty nutrients

Malnutrition has an adverse effect on wound healing. Fatty acids, proteins, carbohydrates, vitamins C, B-complex, A, and the minerals iron, copper, zinc and calcium all play an important part in the healing process (Gray and Cooper 2001). A zinc

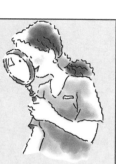

Tips for detecting nutritional problems

Nutritional problems may stem from physical conditions, drugs, diet or lifestyle factors. The list below can help you identify risk factors that make your patient particularly susceptible to nutritional problems.

Physical condition

- Chronic illnesses (such as diabetes) and neurological, cardiac or thyroid problems
- Family history of diabetes or heart disease
- Draining wounds or fistulas
- Weight issues – weight loss of 5% of normal body weight; weight less than 90% of ideal body weight; weight gain or loss of 4.5 kg (10 lb) or more in last 6 months; obesity; or weight gain of 20% above normal body weight
- History of gastrointestinal (GI) disturbances
- Anorexia or bulimia
- Depression or anxiety
- Severe trauma
- Recent chemotherapy or radiation therapy
- Physical limitations, such as paresis or paralysis
- Recent major surgery
- Pregnancy, especially teen or multiple-birth pregnancy.

Drugs and diet

- Fad diets
- Steroid, diuretic or antacid use
- Mouth, tooth or denture problems
- Excessive alcohol intake
- Strict vegetarian diet
- Liquid diet or nil by mouth for more than 3 days.

Lifestyle factors

- Lack of support from family or friends
- Financial problems.

deficiency adversely affects the proliferation phase by slowing the rate of epithelialisation and decreasing the strength of collagen produced – and, thus, the strength of the healing skin. Fatty acids (lipids) are used in cell structures and play a role in the inflammatory process. Collagen synthesis requires protein and zinc plus supplies of carbohydrates and fat. Collagen cross-linking requires adequate amounts of vitamins A, B and C, iron and copper. Vitamin C, iron and zinc are important to developing tensile strength during the maturation phase of wound healing.

The healing process may be enhanced by pre-operative feeding and by the administration of certain nutrients such as glutamine and arginine (Campos *et al.* 2008).

The NICE guidance document *Nutrition Support in Adults* (NICE 2006) offers best practice advice on the care of adults who are malnourished or at risk of malnutrition. This document is available electronically or to order, see page 275 for website.

Protein is a critical component of wound healing. Double up on your patient's protein intake to ensure proper and timely healing.

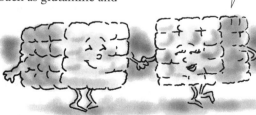

Oxygenation

Wound healing depends on a regular supply of oxygen (Hunt et al. 2004). For example, oxygen is critical for leucocytes to destroy bacteria and for fibroblasts to stimulate collagen synthesis. If the supply is hindered by poor blood flow to the area of the wound or if the patient's ability to take in adequate oxygen is impaired, the result is the same – impaired healing.

Possible causes of inadequate blood flow to the area of the wound include pressure, arterial occlusion or prolonged vasoconstriction, possibly associated with such medical conditions as peripheral vascular disease and atherosclerosis. Possible causes of a lower than necessary systemic blood oxygenation include:

- inadequate oxygen intake
- hypothermia or hyperthermia
- anaemia
- alkalaemia
- other medical conditions, such as chronic obstructive pulmonary disease.

Infection

Infection can be systemic or localised in the wound. A systemic infection, such as pneumonia or tuberculosis, increases the patient's metabolism and thus consumes the fluids, nutrients and oxygen that the body needs for healing.

Damaging developments

A localised infection in the wound itself is more common. Remember, any break in the skin allows bacteria to enter. The infection may occur as part of the injury or may develop later in the healing process. For example, when the inflammatory phase lingers, wound healing is delayed and metabolic by-products of bacterial ingestion accumulate in the wound. This build-up interferes with the formation of new blood vessels and the synthesis of collagen. Infection can also occur in a wound that has been healing normally. This is especially true for larger wounds involving extensive tissue damage. In either case, healing can't progress until the cause of infection is addressed. (See *Recognising infection*, page 40.)

Age

Skin changes that occur with ageing can prolong healing time in elderly patients. Although delayed healing is partially due to physiological changes, it's usually complicated by other problems associated with ageing, such as poor nutrition and hydration, the presence of a chronic condition or the use of multiple medications. (See *Effects of ageing on wound healing*, page 23.)

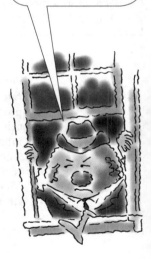

Pay no attention to me! I'm just looking for a way to get under your skin.

Handle with care

Effects of ageing on wound healing

In older adults, the following factors impede wound healing:

- slower turnover rate in epidermal cells
- poorer oxygenation at the wound due to increasingly fragile capillaries and a reduction in skin vascularisation
- altered nutrition and fluid intake resulting from physical changes that can accompany ageing, such as reduced saliva production, a declining sense of smell and taste or decreased stomach motility
- altered nutrition and fluid intake attributable to troubling personal or social issues, such as loose-fitting dentures, financial concerns, eating alone after the death of a spouse or problems preparing or obtaining food
- impaired function of the respiratory or immune systems
- reduced dermal and subcutaneous mass leading to an increased risk of chronic pressure ulcers
- healed wounds that lack tensile strength and are prone to re-injury.

Chronic health conditions

Chronic health conditions such as respiratory disease, diabetes, arthritis and cardiovascular disease can increase the risk of wounds; they can also interfere with systemic and peripheral oxygenation and nutrition, which affect the healing process.

Getting complicated

Impaired circulation, a common problem for patients with diabetes and other disorders, can cause tissue hypoxia (lack of oxygen). Neuropathy associated with diabetes reduces a person's ability to sense pressure. As a result, a diabetic patient may experience trauma, especially to the feet, without realising it. Insulin dependency can impair leucocyte function, which adversely affects cell proliferation.

Hemiplegia and quadriplegia involve the breakdown of muscle tissue and a reduction in the padding around the large bones of the lower body. Because patients with one of these conditions lacks sensation, they are at risk of developing chronic pressure ulcers.

Other conditions that can delay healing include dehydration, end-stage renal disease, thyroid disease, heart failure, peripheral vascular disease and vasculitis and other collagen vascular disorders.

Day and night shifts

Normally, a healthy person shifts position every 15 minutes or so, even during sleep. This prevents tissue damage due to ischaemia. Anything that impairs the ability to sense pressure, including the use

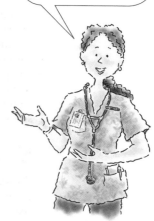

Don't forget that such health problems as respiratory disorders, atherosclerosis, diabetes and malignancies not only increase the risk of wounds but also hinder healing.

of pain medications, spinal cord lesions or cognitive impairment, puts the patient at risk of trauma (the patient can't feel the growing discomfort of pressure and respond to it).

Medications

Any medications that reduce a patient's movement, circulation or metabolic function, such as sedatives or inotropes, have the potential to inhibit their ability to sense and respond to pressure. Also, because movement promotes adequate oxygenation, lack of motion means that peripheral blood delivers less oxygen to the extremities than it should. This is especially problematic for older adults. Remember, oxygen is important; without it, the healing process slows and the potential for complications rises.

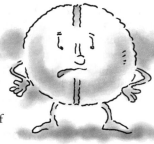

Medications, particularly sedatives, can also cause wound healing complications.

Slow coach

Some medications, such as steroids and chemotherapeutic agents, reduce the body's ability to mount an appropriate inflammatory response. This interrupts the inflammatory phase of healing and can dramatically lengthen healing time, especially in patients with compromised immune systems.

Smoking

Smoking is thought to impact on wound healing in a variety of ways. Toxins contained in cigarette smoke have a particularly damaging effect on the healing process. Hydrogen cyanide, carbon monoxide and nicotine, three key toxins found in cigarette smoke, are believed to cause a number of problems: hydrogen cyanide inhibits oxygen transportation, carbon monoxide binds to haemoglobin in blood in place of oxygen, and nicotine causes vasoconstriction and decreased tissue perfusion (Whiteford 2003). The effect of these toxins significantly reduces the amount of oxygen available for wound healing resulting in potential delays and an increased risk of infection. Smoking just one cigarette can lead to a transient decrease in skin blood flow. Research has shown that postoperative patients who smoke are also at higher risk of a variety of wound-related complications such as infection, wound rupture and necrosis of the wound and flap (Ahn *et al.* 2008). There may also be an impact on wound healing when people are regularly exposed to second-hand smoke (Wong *et al.* 2004).

Socioeconomic factors

Socioeconomic factors can play an important role in determining the patient's ability to concord with a treatment plan. The patient on a fixed income may not be able to afford to make the choice between

A close look at skin layers

Skin is made up of separate layers that function as a single unit. Two distinct layers of skin, the epidermis and dermis, lie above a layer of subcutaneous fatty tissue (sometimes called the *hypodermis*).

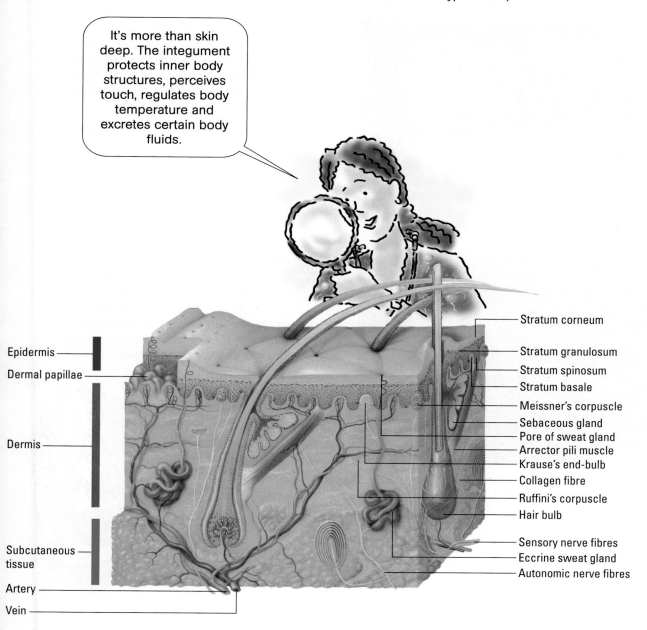

It's more than skin deep. The integument protects inner body structures, perceives touch, regulates body temperature and excretes certain body fluids.

Epidermis

Dermal papillae

Dermis

Subcutaneous tissue

Artery

Vein

Stratum corneum

Stratum granulosum

Stratum spinosum

Stratum basale

Meissner's corpuscle

Sebaceous gland

Pore of sweat gland

Arrector pili muscle

Krause's end-bulb

Collagen fibre

Ruffini's corpuscle

Hair bulb

Sensory nerve fibres

Eccrine sweat gland

Autonomic nerve fibres

Wound bed condition

Wound bed appearance can tell you how well a wound is healing and guide your specific management approach.

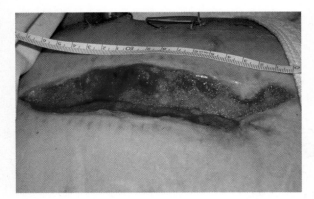

Granulation tissue

When a wound begins to heal, a layer of pale pink granulation tissue covers the wound bed. As this layer thickens, it becomes beefy red. This photo shows a granulation tissue base in an abdominal wound.

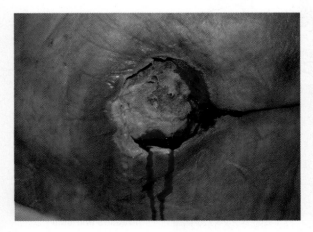

Fibrin slough

Yellow slough or dead tissue on the wound base is usually fibrin left over from the healing process. This slough, or soft necrotic tissue, is a medium for bacteria growth. This photo shows a sacral pressure ulcer with three quarters of the surface area covered with yellow necrotic slough.

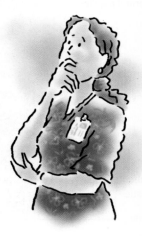

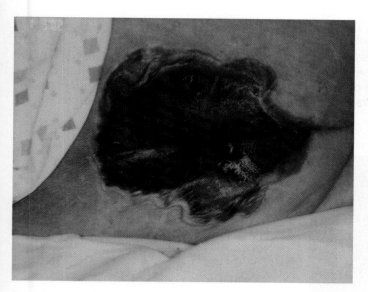

Eschar

Eschar signals necrosis. Dead avascular tissue slows healing and provides a site for microorganisms to proliferate. The photo at left shows a pressure ulcer with eschar; the photo below shows black ischaemic toes.

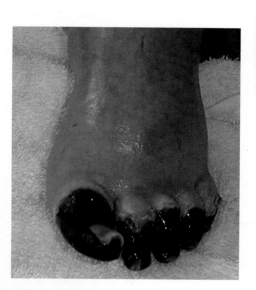

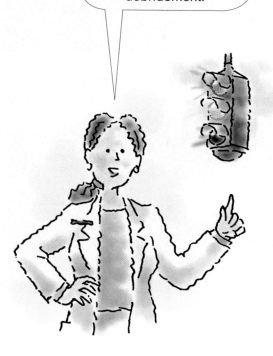

Watch for wound colour signals. Red usually means the wound is healing normally. Yellow means that fibrin is building up and you need to clean the wound. If a wound is black, it needs debridement.

Detecting wound dehiscence

Although surgical wounds typically heal without incident, occasionally the edges of a wound may fail to join or may separate after they begin to heal. This development, called *wound dehiscence*, may lead to evisceration, an even more serious complication in which a portion of a viscous (in an abdominal incision, usually a bowel loop) protrudes through the incision. These photos illustrate a dehisced abdominal wound and a dehisced, healing abdominal incision.

Dehisced abdominal wound (with a colostomy)

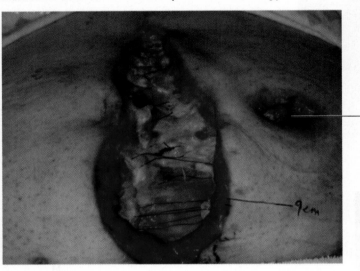

Colostomy

Dehisced, healing abdominal incision

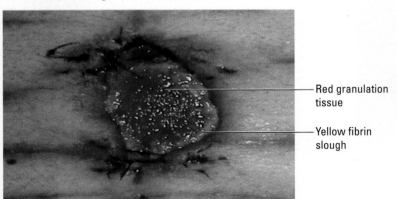

Red granulation tissue

Yellow fibrin slough

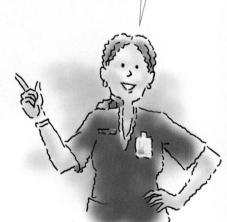

wound treatment, housing and food. If you have a patient who's in this situation, consult social services to determine if alternative payment sources can be found. In time, you may also need to make changes to the treatment plan in order to decrease the patient's costs. Remember to periodically assess the patient for changes in their condition.

Money matters

Income can impact on the patient's living conditions as well. Poor living conditions can influence his ability to heal. It's important to evaluate the patient's home environment and assess its condition and the ability of the patient and their family to manage the wound within that environment.

Working it out

Job loss due to ill-health can also leave a patient without an adequate income. A patient who doesn't have an adequate income may be unable to purchase the necessary wound care supplies, pay for transport to and from appointments or buy healthy and nutritious food. Some people are entitled to free prescriptions but many patients are not; these may be faced with substantial costs related to wound care treatment.

In addition, the patient's work history can influence the risk for disease development such as malignant wounds and venous leg ulceration. It is therefore important to take work history into account when assessing the patient's wound for the first time.

Talk it over

The patient's understanding of their wound treatment is also an important factor in wound management. Ensure that the patient and their carer understand how to manage the wound properly and why advice such as eating and drinking well is important. Always reinforce any verbal instructions given with written information. Written information for patients should be easy to understand (avoiding the use of unecessary jargon and terminology), printed legibly in a plain font, size 12 or above and where appropriate, include simple pictures or diagrams to illustrate the written text. Written information should always include who to contact for further advice on the subject and should be made available in a variety of formats and languages. Further advice on producing written information for patients can be found on the Department of Health website, see page 275.

Cultural cues

Cultural or religious beliefs may prevent the patient from seeking appropriate medical attention or concording with the wound treatment plan. In order to improve the patient's concordance with the plan, evaluate their cultural and religious beliefs to ensure that the treatment plan is in accordance with them.

Psychological factors

The pyschological impact of having a wound is well recognised by experts in the field of wound care but often underestimated by other health professionals and the general public. (For *Psychosocial effects* see Chapter 7, page 151.) Psychological factors have a direct impact on the healing process. Patients who are embarassed by the appearance or smell of their wound may fail to seek help, those who experience unpleasant side-effects of treatment may fail to concord with the treatment plan and anxiety or stress can lead to loss of sleep and reduced appetite.

Such issues can lead to loss of self-esteem and depression. Be sure to provide opportunities for the patient and their carer to discuss their concerns. Support groups can also become an important source of support and encouragement.

Complications of wound healing

The most common complications associated with wound healing are infection, haemorrhage, dehiscence and evisceration.

Infection

Infection is a relatively common complication of wound healing which should be addressed promptly. Infection can delay the healing process, causing the wound to remain static, deteriorate or break down. Infection can spread to surrounding tissues resulting in cellulitus and in some cases, if left untreated, can lead to septicaemia and death. (See *Recognising infection*, page 40.)

Haemorrhage

Internal haemorrhage (bleeding) can result in the formation of a haematoma – a blood clot that solidifies to form a hard lump under the skin. Haematomas are commonly found around bruises.

External haemorrhage is visible bleeding from the wound. External bleeding during healing isn't unusual because the newly developed blood vessels are fragile and rupture easily. This is one reason why a wound needs to be protected by a dressing. However, each time the new blood vessels suffer damage, healing is delayed while repairs are made.

Dehiscence and evisceration

Dehiscence is a separation of the skin and underlying tissue layers. It may occur following surgery, usually between 5 and

Handle with care

Wound healing and the obese patient

The obese patient is at risk for delayed wound healing due to:

- reduced tissue perfusion in adipose tissue and increased tension at the suture line caused by the weight of excess body fat
- excess skin folds (especially if the wound is within one of the folds or if the folds of excess tissue cover a suture line, which may keep the wound moist and allow bacteria to accumulate)
- associated medical conditions such as type 2 diabetes mellitus.

The obese patient is also at increased risk for dehiscence and evisceration because their diet may be seriously lacking in the essential minerals and vitamins that are necessary for proper would healing.

Recognising dehiscence and evisceration

In wound dehiscence, the layers of a wound separate. In evisceration, the viscera (in this case, a bowel loop) protrude through the wound.

Wound dehiscence

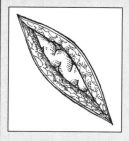

Evisceration of bowel loop

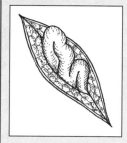

8 days post-operatively (Hunt 1979). Evisceration is similar but involves the protrusion of underlying visceral organs as well. (See *Recognising dehiscence and evisceration*) Dehiscence and evisceration may constitute a surgical emergency, especially if they involve an abdominal wound. If a wound opens without evisceration, it may need to heal by secondary intention. Infection, poor nutrition, advanced age and obesity all increase a patient's risk of dehiscence and evisceration. (See *Wound healing and the obese patient*.)

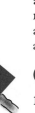

Quick quiz

1. The outermost layer of the skin is the:
   A. epidermis
   B. dermis
   C. hypodermis
   D. subdermal layer.

Answer: A. The epidermis is the outermost layer of the skin. It's composed of epithelial tissue and is supported by the dermis.

2. The layer of skin that contains apocrine sweat glands is the:
   A. stratum corneum
   B. dermis
   C. subcutaneous tissue
   D. stratum basale.

Answer: B. Apocrine glands are situated in the dermis and have ducts that empty into hair follicles.

3.   The structures that deliver oxygen and nutrients to skin cells
are:
    A.   dermatomes
    B.   lymphatics
    C.   capillaries
    D.   quadratics.
Answer: C. A rich network of capillaries delivers oxygen to the
skin's cells.

4.   The main functions of the skin include:
    A.   support, nourishment and sensation
    B.   protection, sensory perception and temperature regulation
    C.   fluid transport, sensory perception and ageing regulation
    D.   support, protection and communication.
Answer: B. The skin's main functions involve protection from
injury, noxious chemicals and bacterial invasion; sensory perception
of touch, temperature and pain; and regulation of body heat.

5.   Which type of wound closes by primary intention?
    A.   second-degree burn
    B.   pressure ulcer
    C.   traumatic injury
    D.   surgical incision.
Answer: D. A surgical incision is an example of a wound that closes
by primary intention, in which there's no deep tissue loss and the
wound edges are well approximated.

6.   Which phase of the wound healing process is responsible for
cleaning the wound and starting the rebuilding process?
    A.   haemostasis
    B.   inflammation
    C.   proliferation
    D.   maturation.
Answer: B. The inflammatory phase is both a defence mechanism
that's vital to preventing infection of the wound and a crucial
component of the healing process.

7.   Which three toxins found in cigarette smoke are particularly
damaging to wounds?
    A. hydrogen cyanide, carbon monoxide and nicotine
    B. hydrogen cyanide, carbon dioxide and oxygen
    C. carbon monoxide, tar and hydrogen cyanide
    D. carbon dioxide, tar and hydrogen.
Answer: A. Hydrogen cyanide inhibits oxygen transportation,
carbon monoxide binds to haemoglobin in blood in place of oxygen,
and nicotine causes vasoconstriction and decreased tissue perfusion.

Scoring

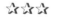 If you answered all seven questions correctly, congratulations! It looks like the information in this chapter has gotten under your skin.

 If you answered five or six questions correctly, good job! It's our sensory perception that you're well healed.

 If you answered fewer than five questions correctly, don't sweat it! After a quick review, this topic won't 'phase' you at all.

References

Ahn, C., Mulligan, P. and Salcido, R.S. (2008) Smoking – the bane of wound healing: biomedical interventions and social influences. *Advances in Skin and Wound Care* 12(5):227–236.

Campos, A.C., Groth, A.K. and Branco, A.B. (2008) Assessment and nutritional aspects of wound healing. *Current Opinion in Clinical Nutrition and Metabolic Care* 11(3):281–288.

Forester, J.C., Zederfeldt, B.H. and Hunt, T.K. (1969) A bioengineering approach to the healing wound. *Journal of Surgical Research* 9:207.

Gray, D. and Cooper, P. (2001) Nutrition and wound healing – what is the link? *Journal of Wound Care* 10(3):86–89.

Holmes, S. (2007) The effects of undernutrition in hospital patients. *Nursing Standard* 22(12):35–38.

Hunt, T.K. (1979) Disorders of repair and their management. In Hunt, T.K. and Dunphy, J.E. (eds). *Fundamentals of Wound Management.* New York: Appleton-Century.

Hunt, T.K., Ellison, E.C. and Sen, C.K. (2004) Oxygen: at the foundation of wound healing – Introduction. *World Journal of Surgery* 28:291–293.

Lindstedt, E. and Sandblom, P. (1975) Wound healing in man: tensile strength of healing wounds in some patient groups. *Annals of Surgery* 181(6):842–846.

Martin, F. (2001) Malnutrition in older people. *Journal of Community Nursing.* 15(08) [on-line] [Accessed on 6 August 2008] Available: http://www.jcn.co.uk/journal.asp?MonthNum=08&YearNum= 2001&Type=backissue&ArticleID=381

National Institute of Health and Clinical Excellence (NICE) (2006) CG32 *Nutrition Support in Adults: Oral Nutrition Support, Enteral Tube Feeding and Parenteral Nutrition.* [on-line] [Accessed on 7 November 2008] Available: http://www.nice.org

Potter, J., Klipstein, K., Reilly, J.J. *et al.* (1995) Nutritional status and clinical course of acute admissions to a geriatric unit. *Age Ageing* 24:131–136.

Whiteford, L. (2003) Nicotine, CO and HCN: the detrimental effects of smoking on wound healing. *British Journal of Community Nursing* 8(12):S22–S26.

Wong, L.S., Green, H.M., Feugate, J.E. *et al.* (2004) Effects of 'second-hand' smoke on structure and function of fibroblasts, cells that are critical for tissue repair and remodelling. *BMC Cell Biology* 5(5):13.

2 Wound assessment and monitoring

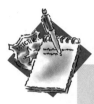

Just the facts

In this chapter, you'll learn:

♦ key elements of assessment
♦ ways to classify wounds according to type, age and depth
♦ accurate documentation of wound progress
♦ tools to track wound healing.

Wound assessment

Each time you assess a wound, remember that you're assessing a patient with a wound – not simply the wound itself. This will help keep you focused on the big picture as you perform your initial assessment and will set the stage for effective monitoring and successful healing.

When you gather information about a wound, you must use all your senses. Be sure to cover the key assessment considerations below as well as assessing the wound bed and exudate levels. As you perform your assessment, remember that it doesn't matter what method you use to record your observations as long as you're consistent.

Key assessment considerations

Several factors influence the body's ability to heal itself, regardless of the type of injury suffered. You should include these elements in your wound assessment:
* cause
* immune status
* blood glucose levels, especially glycosylated haemoglobin (HbA_{1c})

- hydration
- nutrition
- blood albumin and pre-albumin levels
- oxygen and vascular supply
- pain
- psychosocial factors.

Cause

It is essential to consider the cause of the wound when planning care. Ask the patient or carer how and when the wound occurred and consider how the cause may influence the healing process. For example, an injury sustained whilst gardening may be contaminated with soil and will therefore require thorough cleaning and a check for tetanus cover.

Under it all

Where an underlying pathology has caused or contributed to the wound it will be necessary to treat this first to ensure wound healing is not further compromised. For example, a patient presenting with a venous leg ulcer will require compression bandaging to reverse the underlying venous hypertension and patients with diabetes must have their blood glucose levels carefully controlled and any build-up of callus on the foot removed.

Where the wound cause is related to external factors such as direct pressure it will be necessary to remove the factor causing the pressure, for example a hard bed surface, and replace with something more suitable. Failure to treat underlying or contributory causes may delay healing and could result in further wounds developing.

In other words, as you focus on specific wound characteristics and track the healing process; never lose sight of the big picture.

Conflicting theories

You must also be alert to the possibility that the history given by the patient or carer may not be a true representation of what actually happened. If you have any doubts about the real cause of the injury, i.e. if you suspect the wound is a result of non-accidental injury or some other form of abuse, you must refer to your organisation's policy on protection of the vulnerable adult or child immediately.

Immune status

The immune system plays a central role in wound healing. If the patient's immune system is impaired due to disease, such as human immunodeficiency virus (HIV) infection, or as a result of chemotherapy or radiation, you should monitor the wound for impaired healing. Remember, chemotherapeutic agents aren't only used to treat cancer patients; they may also be used to treat inflammatory diseases such as arthritis. Corticosteroids may also depress immune system function.

Blood glucose levels

Blood glucose levels should be below 10 mmol/l (approximately) for satisfactory healing, regardless of the wound's cause. Levels of 10 mmol/l (approximately) or more can impair the function of white blood cells (WBCs), which are important in wound healing because they help prevent infection.

HbA_{1c} is also an indication of glucose control and the efficacy of diabetic therapy. An elevated HbA_{1c} level has the same consequences as an elevated blood glucose level: impaired wound healing and reduced ability to fight infection.

Hydration

Be sure to closely monitor and optimise the patient's hydration status – successful healing depends on it. Skin and subcutaneous tissues need to be well hydrated from the inside. Dehydration impairs the healing process by slowing the body's metabolism. Dehydration also reduces skin turgor, or fullness, leaving skin vulnerable to new wounds.

Nutrition

Nutritional status helps determine the patient's vulnerability to skin breakdown as well as the body's overall ability to heal. A comprehensive assessment of the patient's nutritional status is therefore essential for effective care planning. (See *Parts of a nutritional assessment.*)

Keep in mind that nutrition is complex. If your assessment leads you to believe that the patient's nutritional status places them at risk of skin damage or of delayed wound healing, work with a dietitian to develop the best possible treatment plan.

Blood albumin and pre-albumin levels

Blood albumin and pre-albumin levels are essential factors in wound assessment for two important reasons:
• Skin is primarily constructed of protein, and albumin is a protein. If albumin levels are low, the body lacks an important building block for skin repair.

Parts of a nutritional assessment

A comprehensive nutritional assessment can play an important part in wound care. Remember the four parts of a nutritional assessment, shown here.

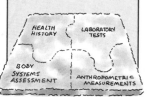

HEALTH HISTORY

LABORATORY TESTS

BODY SYSTEMS ASSESSMENT

ANTHROPOMETRIC MEASUREMENTS

A closer look at albumin

Albumin, a large protein molecule, acts like a magnet to attract water and hold it inside the blood vessel.

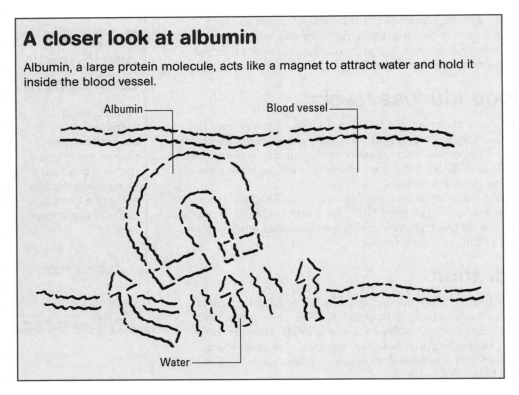

- Albumin is the blood component that provides colloid osmotic pressure – the force that prevents fluid from leaking out of blood vessels into nearby tissues. (See *A closer look at albumin*.) If albumin levels fall below 3.5 g/dl, the patient can develop oedema (fluid leakage into tissues), which compromises wound healing. The patient is also at risk of developing hypotension (low blood pressure) as fluid leaks out of the bloodstream into tissues. If blood pressure falls to the point where adequate blood flow is no longer maintained through the capillaries near the wound, healing slows or stops.

A patient's pre-albumin level may be a better indication of his nutritional status because a normal level (16 to 35 mg/dl) is less affected by liver and renal disease and hydration status than other serum proteins; however, levels can be depressed in inflammatory states independently of nutritional status. Levels should therefore be considered alongside C-reactive protein to differentiate between reduction due to malnutrition or illness (Robinson *et al.* 2003).

Oxygen and vascular supply

Healing requires oxygen – it's that simple. Therefore, anything that impedes full oxygenation also impedes healing. During your assessment, you should consider any factor that may reduce the amount of oxygen available for healing. Possible problems include:

- impaired gas exchange, causing decreased oxygen levels in the blood
- haemoglobin levels too low to transport adequate oxygen
- low blood pressure that fails to drive oxygenated blood through capillaries
- insufficient arterial and capillary supply in the wound area.

Any of these problems on their own or in combination can deprive the wound of the oxygen needed for successful healing.

> Be sure to explain to your patient ways in which smoking cessation facilitates wound healing.

Smoke bomb

Smoking impedes oxygenation of the wound. If the patient is a smoker, explain to them ways in which smoking affects wound healing:

- Nicotine is a powerful vasoconstrictor that narrows peripheral blood vessels, thereby compromising blood flow to the skin.
- Because it's easier for haemoglobin to bind to the carbon monoxide present in cigarette smoke than it is for it to bind to oxygen, the blood that does squeeze through carries far less oxygen than it should.
- Lung tissue damaged by smoke doesn't function as well as it should, resulting in decreased oxygenation.

Pain

In order to promote comfort, you should control the patient's pain to the best of your ability. Pain control also has a practical purpose. In response to pain, the body releases adrenaline (epinephrine), a powerful vasoconstrictor. Vasoconstriction reduces blood flow to the wound. When pain is relieved, vasoconstriction subsides, blood vessels dilate and blood flow to the wound improves.

> If your patient is able, have them rate their pain before and during each dressing change.

Assessing the patient's pain is an important part of wound assessment. You'll want to note pain associated with the injury itself along with pain associated with healing and therapies employed to promote healing. To fully understand the patient's pain, talk with them and ask about their pain. Then, independently, watch to see how they respond to pain and the therapies provided. As always, remember to record your findings. (See *How to assess pain*, page 36.)

Listen and learn

If the patient is conscious and can communicate, have them rate their pain before and during each dressing change. If your notes

How to assess pain

To properly assess your patient's pain, consider the patient's descriptions and your own observations of their reaction to pain and treatments.

Talk to your patient

Begin your pain assessment by asking your patient the following questions:

- Where is the pain located? How long does it last? How often does it occur?
- What does the pain feel like? (Let your patient describe it; don't prompt.)
- What relieves the pain? What makes it worse?
- How do you usually get relief?
- How would you rate your pain on a scale of 0 to 10, with 0 representing no pain and 10 representing the worst pain?

Talking with your patient about their pain in this manner helps them define their pain, for themselves as well as you, and helps you evaluate the effectiveness of therapies used to relieve pain.

Monitor and observe your patient

As you work with your patient, observe their responses to pain and to interventions intended to relieve pain.
Behavioural responses to watch for include:

- altered body position
- moaning
- sighing
- grimacing
- withdrawing from painful stimuli
- crying
- restlessness
- muscle twitching
- immobility.

Sympathetic responses, normally associated with mild-to-moderate pain include:

- pallor
- elevated blood pressure
- dilated pupils
- tension in skeletal muscles
- dyspnoea (shortness of breath)
- tachycardia (rapid heartbeat)
- diaphoresis (sweating).

Parasympathetic responses, which are more common in cases of severe, deep pain include:

- pallor
- lower than normal blood pressure
- bradycardia (slower than normal heartbeat)
- nausea and vomiting
- weakness
- dizziness
- loss of consciousness.

reveal that their pain is higher before the dressing change, it may indicate an impending infection, even before any other signs appear.

If the patient says the dressing change itself is painful, you might consider administering pain medication before the procedure or changing the dressing/procedure technique itself. Remember that wound cleaning has been cited as a key contributory factor in procedure-related pain (Moffatt *et al.* 2002) so take great care when cleaning the wound bed and surrounding skin. It is also important to document all reports or observations of pain and report them to the rest of the team. If the patient's pain isn't documented and communicated they may suffer unnecessary discomfort.

Easy does it

When removing adhered dressings, it is less painful for the patient if you soak the dressing first. Over intact skin, you can also use a silicone-based adhesive remover. Remember to keep the skin taut during removal. Press down on the skin to release the dressing, rather than just pulling the dressing off. Removal in the direction of hair growth will also help minimise discomfort. Sometimes the patient will find it easier to remove the dressing themselves. If the patient still says that dressing removal is painful, reconsider the choice of dressing. Dressings that adhere to the wound bed as well as the surrounding skin can result in tissue trauma as well as unnecessary pain.

Psychosocial factors

Psychosocial factors should be assessed alongside all the factors above. When carrying out the initial patient assessment listen carefully to what your patient does and does not say about the wound and (discreetly) observe their behaviour and body language.

Does your patient:
- Appear anxious or worried about their wound? (e.g. worried about the smell, unable to manage the exudate, can't tolerate the pain)
- Seem low or altered in mood? (e.g. fed up, tearful, angry)
- Express resentful or guilty feelings? (e.g. Why me?, Is it my fault?)
- Seem discouraged or pessimistic about progress to date? (e.g. can't see that it will get better, doesn't feel treatment is working)
- Describe a change in social habits (e.g. staying at home, losing touch with friends, refusing visitors)
- Describe a change in personal habits (e.g. appearance, dress, hygiene, reduced appetite)

Psychosocial factors are also about lifestyle, environmental and family concerns. Ask your patient about their normal daily activities, their hobbies and interests. A patient who loves their daily dog walk may become very unhappy if their leg ulcer makes it too painful to walk far; analgesia and a different bandage system may help. The patient who loves television but cannot sit for long periods because of their pressure ulcer may be grateful for a portable television in their bedroom. The patient who feels very isolated as a result of their fungating tumour may appreciate family and friends helping with the shopping and organising a visiting rota.

Remember, you are trying to assess how the wound is affecting your patient and how they feel about having it. This will help you plan the right care for them. This might include giving reassurance about their progress, education about the wound, advice on support groups or clubs in the area or referral for financial or employment advice. It may include referral to a specialist for further help or assessment, e.g. a psychologist or a social worker.

Assessing the wound

Assess the wound and the surrounding skin only after they have been cleaned. As you assess the wound, record information about:
- appearance of wound bed (tissue types)
- appearance of wound margins
- surrounding skin.
- dimensions including tunnelling and undermining
- presence of moisture.

Appearance of wound bed (tissue types)

The appearance of the wound and type of tissue in the wound bed provides important information about the wound and how it's healing. The tissue types seen are granulation, slough, necrotic and epithelial.

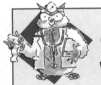

Get wise to wounds

What's missing?

If wound photography is a routine part of your wound documentation system, remember that a picture may be worth a thousand words but your assessment skills and clinical observations are still essential. Many wound characteristics can't be recorded accurately – or at all – on film. These include:

- location
- depth
- tunnel measurement
- odour
- feel of surrounding tissue
- pain.

   All of this information is needed if the healthcare team is to make sound treatment decisions.

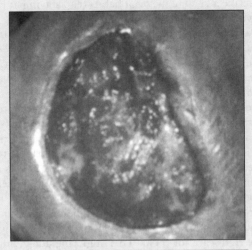

Photograph reprinted with permission from the National Pressure Ulcer Advisory Panel slide series #1. Available: www.npuap.org.

Granulation tissue

In a full-thickness wound, healthy, moist, red/pink granulation tissue is a sign of healing. Healthy granulation tissue is soft with a slightly granular (bumpy) surface. If you note very smooth red tissue in a partial-thickness wound, it's most likely to be the dermis. In a full-thickness wound, it's probably muscle tissue – not granulation tissue. Factors such as tissue oxygenation, tissue hydration, infection and nutrition can alter the colour and quality of granulation tissue.

Slough tissue

You may also see 'slough' in the wound bed. True slough is a yellowish, creamy tissue comprising debris from the healing process such as dead WBCs produced as a by-product of the inflammatory process. It is usually soft in texture and may or may not be firmly adhered to the wound bed. Some practitioners also use the term 'slough' to describe liquefying necrotic tissue which presents as grey/black/brown stringy through to softer semi-liquid matter.

A very small amount of slough will not impede healing to any great degree but anything more will require removal through application of appropriate dressings. (See Chapter 4, *Wound care products*.) It is important to distinguish between slough and tendon which may appear similar in appearance to the inexperienced practitioner.

Necrotic tissue

There may also be necrotic (dead) tissue in the wound bed. This is sometimes referred to as eschar or non-viable tissue. This tissue is black or black–brown in colour, usually dry in texture and must be removed for healing to progress. Areas of necrotic or devitalised tissue may mask underlying damage, abscesses and collections of fluid. Leaving necrotic tissue in the wound bed may result in infection (as the necrotic tissue can act as a source of nutrition for bacteria) and may prevent granulation tissue forming in the wound bed. Both of these situations will stop the wound progressing successfully. Removal of necrotic tissue can be achieved by application of appropriate dressings (see Chapter 4, *Wound care products*) or by skilled debridement (see Chapter 3, *Debridement*, page 74). Take care though, some necrotic tissue such as the dry gangrene seen in some diabetic foot ulcers should be left in place due to the additional demands that removing it puts on the impaired blood supply (see *Diabetic foot ulcers*, page 197).

Epithelial tissue

In the final stage of the proliferative phase of healing, when the wound bed has filled with granulation tissue, new epithelial cells cover the surface of the wound to complete closure. This fragile new tissue is pale pinkish/white in appearance and appears at the wound margins and around the base of the hair follicles before spreading across the wound surface. The wound bed should still be moist at this stage, if the wound dries out the process of epithelialisation will be impaired. Healthy wounds will have epithelial tissue that appears almost flush with the wound surface, wounds that are in a non-healing state tend to have steep epithelial edges.

The presence of different tissue types in the wound bed should be recorded and an estimation made of the percentage amount of each.

Recognising infection

Early recognition of the signs of infection is important to prevent unnecessary delays in healing and prolonged patient distress. All open wounds will be contaminated to some extent by microorganisms although these do not usually cause a delay in healing. If wound bed conditions enable the microbes to multiply they will colonise the wound bed but, again, they will not usually cause delays in healing. If colonisation becomes overly burdensome to the wound it will eventually cause a host reaction and infection will be established. In infected wounds, microorganisms multiply and invade host tissue causing an overt immunological reaction. At this point wound healing is disrupted. Sometimes the stage just before infection is referred to as critical colonisation, when the wound is almost but not quite overcome by bacteria. This stage is difficult to detect clinically. If suspected, swift preventative action such as the use of topical antimicrobial dressings may prevent a full blown infection establishing.

Indicators on

The 'classic' clinical indicators of infection are erythema (redness), heat, oedema (swelling), pain and pus although signs of infection can vary from wound to wound and between different bacterial species. Chronic wounds often present somewhat differently to acute wounds. The following are considered important indicators of wound infection in chronic wounds (Cutting 1998):

- abscess
- cellulitus
- abnormal discharge (purulent, haemopurulent, high levels of exudate, high viscosity)
- elevated body temperature
- friable tissue (fragile, bleeds easily)
- pocketing at base of wound
- malodour
- wound breakdown.

If the wound is failing to progress and shows one or more of the clinical indicators of infection, consider sending a wound swab or exudate sample for culturing. Swab results may give some indication of organisms involved in the infection but reliability is relatively poor when compared to exudate samples which enable microbiology staff to give more accurate results. Ideally, obtain a swab or bottled sample of the clear fluid expressed from the wound tissue after you've thoroughly cleaned the wound. This is more likely to produce a sample of the bacteria in question. Tissue biopsies are even better, usually providing accurate information regarding the type of organisms involved in the infection and enabling the right antibiotic therapy to be commenced, however, tissue biopsies are not carried out routinely as they are invasive and must be carried out by a suitably trained healthcare professional. (See *Infection*, page 146.)

For further information on identifying infection see the European Wound Management Association (EWMA) position document *Identifying criteria for wound infection*, see page 275 for website.

Appearance of wound margins

Wound margins can indicate the stage of healing and provide important clues as to the wound aetiology. When assessing wound margins, you'll want to see skin that's smooth – not rolled – and firmly adhered to the wound bed.

Margins that are rolled under may indicate wound bed desiccation (drying out) whilst loose skin at the edges may indicate additional shearing injury (separation of skin layers), possibly due to a rough transfer or repositioning. Increased moisture levels in the wound bed and improved transfer and repositioning techniques should prevent recurrence.

Steep margins and a 'punched-out' ulcer, are often associated with arterial ulceration whereas outwardly rolling margins may be suggestive of malignancy. Discoloured margins can indicate unusual aetiologies such as pyoderma gangrenosum, although this is more difficult to determine in darker skin. In both these cases, referral for specialist advice is essential.

Surrounding skin

The appearance and condition of the surrounding skin is as important as that of the wound bed.

The condition of the surrounding skin can alert you to problems that can impede healing:
• Dry, flaky, itchy skin (sometimes with evidence of scratching) may indicate eczema which will need allergen-free emollients and possibly referral for dermatology opinion. If the problem is limited to just a little dryness, the skin can be moisturised with an emollient or cream. All moisturisers should be applied following the direction of hair growth to avoid follicular irritation.

- Whitish, spongy, soft skin indicates maceration, due to excess moisture, and signals the need for a protective barrier around the wound and a more absorbent dressing.
- Red skin can indicate inflammation, injury (for example, tape burn, excessive pressure or chemical exposure), or infection. Remember that inflammation is only healthy during the inflammatory phase of healing. If redness is difficult to determine due to skin colour, feel for the warmth of inflammation using the back of the hand.
- Purple skin can indicate bruising – a sign of trauma, deep tissue injury or clotting problems. Remember, discoloration shows more readily on lighter skin tones; in darker skin, colour changes may be difficult to detect. A careful history and close inspection will help. Do not forget, wherever bruising occurs the possibility of non-accidental injury or abuse must be considered.

> If your patient's wound is surrounded by white skin, suspect maceration; if you observe purple skin, suspect bruising.

Let your fingers do the talking

During your assessment of the area around the wound, use your fingers and backs of your hands to gain valuable information. For example, gently probe the tissue around the wound bed to determine if it's soft or hard (indurated). Indurated tissue, even in the absence of erythema (redness), is one indication of infection. Similarly, if the patient has dark skin, it may be impossible to see colour cues. Again, your fingers can help. Probe the area around the wound bed and compare the feel to surrounding healthy skin. A tender area of skin that appears shiny and feels hard may indicate inflammation.

The back of the hand can be used to assess the skin temperature; the skin should feel warm to touch (depending on the room temperature), coolness may indicate ischaemia and heat may indicate inflammation or infection.

Dimensions
Get out your ruler

The most common method of measuring wound dimensions is to use a tape measure. Make sure it's a disposable device to prevent contamination and cross-contamination. Record the length of the wound as the longest overall distance across the wound (regardless of orientation), and record the width as the longest measurement perpendicular (at a right angle) to your length measurement. (See *Measuring a wound*, page 43.)

> Use a cm² tracing grid or disposable ruler to measure your patient's wound.

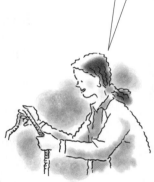

Get wise to wounds

Measuring a wound

When measuring a wound, first determine the longest distance across the open area of the wound – regardless of orientation. In this photo, note the line used to illustrate length.

A wound's width is simply the longest distance across the wound at a right angle to the length. Note the relationship of length and width in this photo. Measure and record areas of reddened, intact skin and white skin as surrounding erythema and maceration – not as part of the wound itself. For a wound like the one in this photo, you would also record a depth and note any areas of tunnelling or undermining. Length × width can be a useful marker of wound size but do not use it to calculate surface area, it will not be accurate!

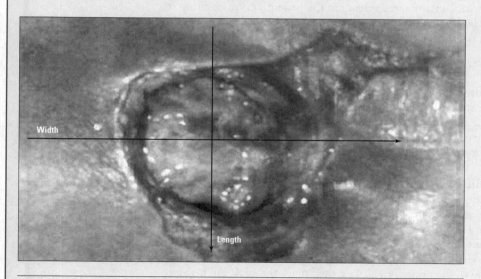

Photograph reprinted with permission from Ayello, E.A. and Baranoski, S. Wound Care Essentials: Practice Principles. Philadelphia: Lippincott Williams & Wilkins, 2004.

Be sure to record any observed areas of intact skin discoloration around the wound opening separately – not as part of the wound bed. Record all measurements in centimetres (cm) and mark on a wound diagram which points have been used for which measurements. Remember though, if you multiply your length × breadth measurements to find the surface area of the wound, you will have a result that overestimates the true size (unless you have a nice neat rectangular wound!).

Just a trace

A more accurate way to measure the wound size is to use wound tracing. Wound margins are traced onto a sheet of clear plastic with a cm^2 grid printed on it; a disposable backing ensures the tracing sheet remains uncontaminated during the procedure. You can use the tracing to calculate an approximate wound area by counting the number of full and partial squares contained in the wound circumference. This method is simple and fairly quick. It is important, however, that the pen nib used to do the tracing is not too thick and that all assessors trace the wound margins from the same starting point to minimise error, also be careful not to cause your patient any discomfort by pressing on the wound when tracing. Retain the uncontaminated tracing in the patient's notes ensuring it is clearly labelled with the patient's name and the date and remember to dispose of the contaminated backing into a clinical waste bag.

How deep

To measure wound depth, you'll need a sterile flexible foam-tipped device or wound swab. Gently insert the device into the deepest portion of the wound and then carefully mark the stick where it meets the edge of the skin. Remove the device and measure the distance from your mark to the end to determine depth.

Tunnelling and undermining

It's also important to measure tunnels, or sinus tracts (extensions of the wound bed into adjacent tissue), and undermining (areas of the wound bed that extend under the skin). Measure tunnelling and undermining just as you would wound depth. Carefully insert a sterile flexible foam-tipped device to the bottom of the tunnel or to the end of the undermined area; then mark the stick and measure the distance from your mark to the end of the device. If a tunnel is large, palpate it with a gloved finger rather than a foam-tipped device because you can sense the end of the tunnel better with your finger. This also minimises the risk of damaging the tissue.

What a picture

Because accurately recording wound dimensions and wound bed appearance is important, many healthcare facilities use photography as a tool in wound assessment. If photography is available in your clinical area, it should be included in your assessment of wound characteristics. Some photographic techniques produce a picture with a grid overlay that's useful for measuring, or sometimes a disposable paper ruler is placed in the photograph alongside the wound. When taking wound photographs you should follow your local policies and guidelines for obtaining consent and ensuring privacy and dignity are maintained. These should include maintenance of privacy during the procedure, protecting the identity of the patient in the photograph wherever possible and ensuring labelling of photographs is restricted to hospital number rather than name. Photographs should never be used for any purpose other than that for which consent has been obtained. The Department of Health gives clear guidance on gaining consent for photography (Department of Health 2001).

Storage methods and access rights should also be considered, particularly if the images are digital. Digital images must be stored in a secure location on a password protected computer. It is not appropriate to take images with a mobile phone where the potential for accidental release to a wider audience exists. Remember also that there are many qualities of the wound that a camera simply can't record. (See *What's missing?*, page 38.)

Moisture (exudate)

The wound bed should be moist – but not overly moist. Moisture allows the cells and chemicals needed for healing to move about the wound surface. In acute wounds, moisture (or exudate) is produced as a normal by-product of the inflammatory process. It contains a variety of substances essential to healing, such as growth factors, nutrients and leucocytes (Thomas 1997). The importance of moisture in the promotion of wound healing has long been recognised (Winter 1962).

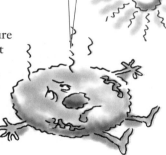

Gasp! Dryness is a drag. If the wound bed is too dry, I can't move. This makes it hard for me to advance healing.

Desert storm

In dry wound beds, cells involved in healing, which normally exist in a fluid environment, can't move. WBCs can't fight infection, enzymes such as collagenase can't break down dead material, and macrophages can't carry away debris. The wound edges curl up to preserve the moisture that remains in the edge and epithelial cells (new skin cells) fail to grow over and cover the wound. Healing grinds to a halt and necrotic tissue builds up.

Flood watch

Too much exudate poses a different problem. It floods the wound and spills out onto the skin, where the constant moisture causes maceration. Maceration, seen as sponge-like, moist, whitish, tissue is difficult to reverse and can result in increased wound size and cell death. Also, in non-healing (chronic) wounds, the composition of exudate changes from that seen in acute wounds. In particular, the high levels of matrix metalloproteinases (naturally occurring enzymes which actively destroy proteins) can cause considerable damage by destroying healthy tissue (Baker and Leaper 2000).

Possible indicators of proteinase damage include:
- Discoloration of the wound bed
- Excoriation at the wound margins and surrounding skin
- Pain in and around the wound
- A delay in pace of healing.

For further information on exudate composition, assessment and management, refer to the World Union of Wound Healing Societies consensus document on Wound Exudate, see page 275 for website.

Assessing exudate

To begin collecting information about wound exudate, inspect the dressing as you remove it and record answers to questions, such as:
- Is the drainage well contained or is it oozing from the edges? If it's oozing, consider using a more absorbent dressing or increase the frequency of dressing change.
- If you're using an occlusive dressing, were the dressing edges well sealed? If the patient has faecal incontinence, it's even more important to note the seal status.
- Is the dressing saturated or dry?
- How much exudate is there: a scant, moderate or large amount?*
- What is the colour of the exudate? (See Chapter 8, *Exudate*, page 189.)
- Is the exudate malodorous?
- What is the consistency of the exudate: watery, viscous?

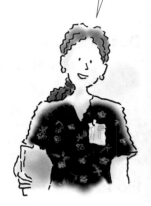

Remember to document the colour, amount, consistency and odour of wound exudate.

Consistency

Consider the consistency of the wound exudate or drainage. If it has a thick, creamy texture, the wound contains an excessive amount of bacteria; however, this doesn't necessarily mean a clinically significant infection is present. Exudate might be creamy because it contains WBCs that have killed bacteria. The exudate is also contaminated with surface bacteria that naturally live in moist environments on the human body. Because of this normal bacterial colonisation, it is important to only use swab cultures when clinical indicators of infection are present.

Malodour

If kept clean, a non-infected wound usually produces little odour. (One exception is the odour present under some hydrocolloid

---

*Assessing the volume of wound exudate is usually subjective unless it is being collected in a wound drainage bag or canister. It may help to use the dressing wear time as a guide to how much exudate is being produced.

Get wise to wounds

Drainage descriptors

This chart provides terminology that you can use to describe the colour and consistency of wound drainage.

Description	Colour and consistency
Serous	• Clear or light yellow • Thin and watery
Sanguineous	• Red (with fresh blood) • Thin
Serosanguineous	• Pink to light red • Thin and watery
Purulent	• Creamy yellow, green, white or tan • Thick and opaque

dressings that develops as a by-product of the degradation process.) A newly detected malodour (offensive or bad smell) might be a sign of infection. Be sure to record your findings and report them to the rest of the team. When documenting wound malodour, it's important to include when you noted it and whether it went away with wound cleaning. Malodour odour that remains after wound cleaning may indicate infection. Several bacteria such as *Pseudomonas* sp. produce a very distinctive odour which can be helpful in determining the colonising organisms.

If malodour develops, it can present an embarrassing or otherwise uncomfortable situation for the patient as well as his family, guests and room-mate. If you notice a malodour, or if the patient says he notices one, use a malodour management dressing (see Chapter 4, *Wound care products*) and a malodour eliminator. Malodour eliminators differ from air fresheners because they aren't scents that mask bad smells but rather compounds that bind with, and neutralise, the molecules responsible for the malodour.

Wound classification

The words you choose to describe your observations of a specific wound have to communicate the same thing to other members of the healthcare team, the patient's family and, ultimately, the

Get wise to wounds

Tailoring wound care to wound assessment

Tissue type	Management techniques
Granulation tissue	• Cover the wound to keep it clean and protected. Keep the wound moist. • For minimal exudate, use a transparent film, hydrocolloid or hydrogel dressing. • For excess exudate use foams, alginates or hydrofibres to absorb the excess drainage. • Remember, beefy red may indicate bioburden of the wound bed and a topical antimicrobial may be warranted (silver, cadexomer iodine).
Fibrin slough	• Use a moisture retentive dressing such as a hydrogel or hydrocolloid to stimulate autolytic debridement (separation of slough from the wound bed) such as transparent films, hydrocolloids or hydrogels OR use an alginate or hydrofibre to absorb excess exudate and support autolytic debridement OR consider using larvae therapy (bio-surgery) for a quicker result. • Consider topical antimicrobials if infection indicated.
Eschar	• Depending on the wound type and the patient's suitability for anaesthesia use surgical debridement or sharp debridement at the bedside (only with appropriate qualification and training) OR use a moisture retentive dressing to stimulate autolytic debridement such as transparent films, hydrocolloids or hydrogels. • Keep wounds with inadequate blood supply clean and dry. • Topical antimicrobials may also be indicated in this type of wound as the tissue begins to break down.

patient themselves. This is a tall order when you consider that even wound care experts debate the descriptive phrases they use. Slough or eschar? Undermining or tunnelling? How much exudate is 'moderate'? Is the colour green or yellow?

A useful way to classify wounds is to use the basic system described here, which focuses on three categories of fundamental characteristics:

- type
- age
- depth.

Type

Two basic types of wounds exist: surgical and non-surgical. A surgical wound is caused by a surgical procedure. A non-surgical wound can be caused by trauma or may be a pressure ulcer, diabetic foot ulcer or vascular ulcer, for example. (See *Tailoring wound care to wound assessment*.)

Age

When determining wound age, you need to first determine if the wound is acute or non-healing (chronic). However, this determination can present a problem if you adhere solely to a timeline. For instance, just how long is it before an acute wound becomes a chronic wound?

A different way of thinking

Rather than base your determination solely on time, consider a wound acute if it's new or making progress as expected. Consider a wound chronic if it isn't healing in a timely fashion. The main idea is that, in a chronic wound, healing has slowed or stopped and the wound is no longer getting smaller and shallower. Even if the wound bed appears healthy, red and moist, if healing fails to progress, consider it a chronic wound.

More bad than good

Chronic wounds don't heal as easily as acute wounds. The exudate in chronic wounds contains a greater amount of destructive enzymes (matrix metalloproteinases), and fibroblasts (the cells that function as the architects in wound healing) seem to lose their 'oomph'. They're less effective at producing collagen, divide less often and send fewer signals to other cells telling them to divide and fill the wound. In other words, the wound changes from one that's vigorous and ready to heal, to one that's downright lazy!

Depth

Depth is another fundamental characteristic used to classify wounds. In your assessment, record wound depth as partial-thickness or full-thickness. (See *Classifying wound depth*, page 50.)

Partial-thickness

Partial-thickness wounds normally heal quickly because they involve only the epidermal layer of the skin or extend through the epidermis into (but not through) the dermis. The dermis remains at least partially intact to generate the new epidermis needed to close the wound. Partial-thickness wounds are also less susceptible to infection because part of the body's first level of defence (partial dermis) is still intact. These wounds tend to be painful, however, and need protection from the air to reduce pain as well as speed healing.

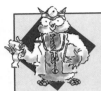

Get wise to wounds

Classifying wound depth

A wound is classified as partial-thickness or full-thickness according to its depth. Partial-thickness wounds involve only the epidermis or extend into the dermis but not through it. Full-thickness wounds extend through the dermis into tissues beneath and may expose adipose tissue, muscle or bone. These diagrams illustrate the relative depth of both classifications.

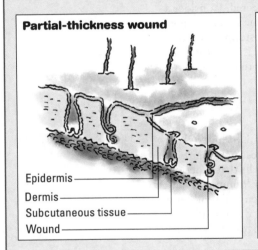

Partial-thickness wound

Epidermis
Dermis
Subcutaneous tissue
Wound

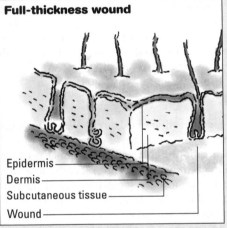

Full-thickness wound

Epidermis
Dermis
Subcutaneous tissue
Wound

Full-thickness

Full-thickness wounds penetrate completely through the skin into underlying tissues. The wound may expose adipose tissue (fat), muscle, tendon or bone. In the abdomen, you may see adipose tissue or omentum (the covering of the bowel). If the omentum is penetrated, the bowel may protrude through the wound (evisceration). Granulation tissue may be visible if the wound has started to heal.

Full-thickness wounds heal by granulation and contraction, which require more body resources and more time than the healing of partial-thickness wounds. When assessing a full-thickness wound, report its depth as well as its surface area, length and width.

The added pressure of pressure ulcers

In the case of pressure ulcers, wound depth allows you to stage or grade the ulcer. (See Chapter 8, *Pressure ulcers*.)

Wound monitoring

The picture of the wound that you paint during your initial assessment plays an important role in wound monitoring.

Monitor the patient throughout the healing process, periodically reassessing the wound status and documenting its progress towards full healing.

Paint a picture

Your initial assessment sets the benchmark for subsequent monitoring and reassessment activities. One assessment is a static report; a series of assessments, however, can illustrate the dynamic aspect of the healing process. In this way, all members of the

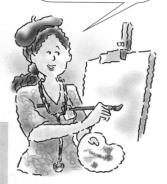

Memory jogger

Use the mnemonic device WOUND PICTURE to help you recall and organise key facts in your documentation:

Wound or ulcer location

Odour (in the room or after uncovering the wound)

Ulcer category, stage (for pressure ulcer) or classification (for diabetic ulcer) and depth (partial-thickness or full-thickness)

Necrotic tissue

Dimension (shape, length, width, depth); drainage colour, consistency and amount (scant, moderate, large)

Pain (when it occurs, what relieves it, patient's description and patient's rating on scale of 0 to 10)

Induration (hard or soft surrounding tissue)

Colour of wound bed (red–yellow–black or combination)

Tunnelling (length and direction – towards patient's right, left, head, feet)

Undermining (length and direction, using clock references to describe)

Redness or other discoloration in surrounding skin

Edge of skin loose or tightly adhered and edges flat or rolled under.

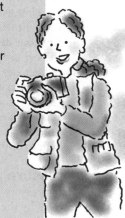

healthcare team can see the patient's progress towards healing (or failure to heal), developing complications and the relative success of interventions. The view will depend on the accuracy, quality and consistency of your documentation.

In the course of a wound assessment, you will amass a lot of useful information about the patient, his environment, the characteristics of his wound and his current status in the healing process. When documenting your assessment, be sure to include the date and time of your observations. Also, strive to obtain accurate measurements, using appropriate units of measurement. Make sure that the entire healthcare team is using the same tool to measure the patient's wound. Remember to document only the facts, not your opinions about the wound. The Nursing and Midwifery Council provides an advice sheet on record keeping, see page 275 for website.

The prospect of monitoring, reassessing and documenting over time may seem daunting; however, several good wound assessment tools are available to help you – or your clinical area may have its own.

Wound assessment tools

Wound assessment tools are designed to encourage a systematic approach to assessment. A good tool will therefore include all the key assessment parameters (as previously described) essential to a comprehensive, holistic wound assessment. An accurately completed assessment will provide evidence of care given and enable you to justify your decision making if called into question at a later date.

There are many wound assessment tools in use, most of which have been designed with a specific clinical setting in mind. It is important to choose a tool that works for the patients in your setting, i.e. the needs of a patient in a leg ulcer clinic will differ to those of a child in a paediatric unit. Although, where possible, the use of the same tool across care settings is recommended in order to enhance communication between professionals in different areas.

Pressure ulcer scale for healing

The pressure ulcer scale for healing (PUSH) tool was developed and revised by the National Pressure Ulcer Advisory Panel (NPUAP) in the US and is only applicable to pressure ulcers. It's simple, quick and easy to score. (See *PUSH tool*, page 53.)

When working with this tool, you develop three scores: one for the surface area (length × width), one for the drainage amount and one for the tissue type in the wound during each review. The sum of these scores yields a total score for the wound on a given day.

PUSH tool

The Pressure Ulcer Scale for Healing (PUSH) tool is simple to use and quick and easy to score.

Patient name *Doris McCoy*   User location *Rockdale Nursing Home*

Patient I.D. # *0162386*   Date *26 July 2006*

Directions

Observe and measure the pressure ulcer. Categorise the ulcer with respect to surface area, exudate and type of wound tissue. Record a subscore for each of the ulcer characteristics. Add the subscores to obtain the total score. A comparison of total scores measured over time provides an indication of the improvement or deterioration in pressure ulcer healing.

Length × width	0 0 cm²	1 < 0.3 cm²	2 0.3 to 0.6 cm²	3 (0.7 to 1 cm²)	4 1.1 to 2 cm²	5 2.1 to 3 cm²	Subscore 3
	6 3.1 to 4 cm²	7 4.1 to 8 cm²	8 8.1 to 12 cm²	9 12.1 to 24 cm²	10 > 24 cm²		
Exudate amount	0 None	1 Light	2 (Moderate)	3 Heavy			Subscore 2
Tissue type	0 Closed	1 (Epithelial tissue)	2 Granulation tissue	3 Slough	4 Necrotic tissue		Subscore 1
						Total score:	6

Length × width

Measure the greatest length (head-to-toe) and the greatest width (side-to-side) using a centimetre ruler. Multiply these two measurements (length × width) to obtain an estimate of surface area in cm². Don't guess! Always use a centimetre ruler and always use the same method each time the ulcer is measured.

Exudate amount

Estimate the amount of exudate (drainage) present after removing the dressing and before applying any topical agent to the ulcer. Estimate the exudate as none, light, moderate or heavy.

Tissue type

This refers to the types of tissue that are present in the wound (ulcer) bed. Score as a 4 if you note necrotic tissue. Score as a 3 if you observe slough but no necrotic tissue. Score as a 2 if the wound is clean and contains granulation tissue. Score a superficial wound that's re-epithelialising as a 1. When the wound is closed, score it as a 0. The following guidelines describe each tissue type:

4 – Necrotic tissue (eschar): Black, brown or tan tissue that adheres firmly to the wound bed or ulcer edges and may be either firmer or softer than surrounding tissue

3 – Slough: Yellow or white tissue that adheres to the ulcer bed in strings or thick clumps or is mucinous

2 – Granulation tissue: Pink or beefy red tissue with a shiny, moist, granular appearance

1 – Epithelial tissue: For superficial ulcers, new pink or shiny tissue (skin) that grows in from the edges or as islands on the ulcer surface

0 – Closed or resurfaced: Completely covered wound with epithelium (new skin)

Adapted with permission from PUSH tool version 3.0, © 1998 National Pressure Ulcer Advisory Panel, Reston, Va.

This score is then plotted on a pressure ulcer healing record and healing graph. By recording and reviewing scores over time, you can determine the pace of progress towards healing.

Wound Healing Scale

The wound healing scale is a simple classification system that combines a designation for wound stage, or thickness, with a tissue descriptor. Using this tool, you can track the general direction of healing by noting, for example, that this week the wound is an FG (full-thickness with granulation tissue), whereas last week it was an FN (full-thickness with necrotic tissue). The tool can be used for all types of wounds, although it was developed initially for use with pressure ulcers.

The Bates-Jensen wound assessment tool

The Bates-Jensen tool (Sussman and Bates-Jensen 2006) lists key wound assessment criteria and uses a numerical scoring system to chart the wounds progress or otherwise. Criteria include wound size, depth, different tissue types and presence of induration in surrounding tissue. Each criterion is sub-divided into categories which are given a score. For example, 'depth' is sub-divided into non-blanchable erythema on intact skin (1), partial-thickness skin loss involving epidermis and/or dermis (2), full-thickness skin loss involving damage or necrosis of subcutaneous tissue (3), obscured by necrosis (4) and full-thickness skin loss with extensive destruction, tissue necrosis or damage to muscle, bone or supporitng structures (5). Wound healing progress is plotted on a wound status continuum at each evaluation. The tool is particularly useful for open, non-healing wounds.

Recognising complications

It's important to monitor and track, or reassess, wound status to identify signs and symptoms of complications or failure to heal as early in the process as possible. Early intervention improves the likelihood of resolving complications successfully and getting the healing process back on track.

Seeing is believing

You'll conduct your reassessments using the same criteria used in the initial assessment, with one added advantage – perspective. Careful monitoring can help you catch failure to heal early so you can intervene appropriately. (See *Recognising failure to heal*, pages 55–56.)

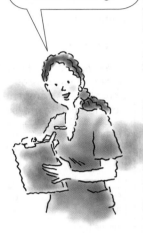

Use the PUSH tool for a quick and easy way to document pressure ulcer healing.

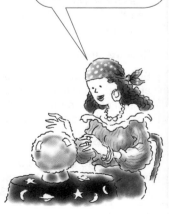

In wound care, you may be able to foresee problems by recognising signs of complications or failure to heal.

Get wise to wounds

Recognising failure to heal

This chart presents the most common signs of failure to heal as well as associated probable causes and appropriate interventions.

Sign	Causes	Interventions
Wound bed		
Too dry	• Exposure of tissue and cells normally in a moist environment to air • Inadequate hydration	• Add moisture regularly. • Use a dressing that retains moisture, such as a transparent film, hydrocolloid or hydrogel dressing.
No change in size or depth for 2 weeks	• Pressure or trauma to the area • Poor nutrition, poor circulation, or inadequate hydration • Poor control of disease processes such as diabetes • Inadequate pain control • Infection	• Reassess the patient for local or systemic problems that impair wound healing, and intervene as necessary.
Increase in size or depth	• Ischaemia due to excess pressure or poor circulation • Infection	• Poor circulation may not be resolvable, but consider adding warmth to the area and administering a vasodilator or antiplatelet medication. Address possible infection.
Necrosis	• Ischaemia	• Consider performing debridement if the remaining living tissue has adequate circulation.
Increase in drainage or change of drainage colour from clear to purulent	• Autolytic or larvae debridement • Infection	• If caused by autolytic or larvae debridement, no intervention is necessary. An increase in drainage or change of drainage colour is expected because of the breakdown of dead tissue. • If debridement isn't the cause, assess the wound for infection.

(continued)

Recognising failure to heal *(continued)*

Sign	Causes	Interventions
Wound bed		
Tunnelling	• Pressure over bony prominences • Presence of foreign body • Deep infection	• Protect the area from pressure. • Irrigate and inspect the tunnel as carefully as possible for a hidden suture or leftover bit of dressing material. • If the tunnel doesn't shorten in length each week, thoroughly clean and obtain a tissue biopsy for infection and, with a chronic wound, for possible malignancy.
Wound edges		
Red, hot skin; tenderness; and induration	• Inflammation due to excess pressure or infection	• Protect the area from pressure. • If pressure relief doesn't resolve the inflammation within 24 hours, topical antimicrobial therapy may be indicated.
Maceration (white skin)	• Excess moisture	• Protect the skin with a non-sting barrier film. • Use a more absorptive dressing, ensure correct size is used.
Rolled skin edges	• Too-dry wound bed	• Use a moisture-retentive dressing to rehydrate the wound. • If rolling isn't resolved in 1 week, debridement of the edges may be necessary.
Undermining or ecchymosis of surrounding skin (loose or bruised skin edges)	• Excess shearing force to the area	• Initiate measures to protect the area, especially during patient transfers.

The sooner, the better

Success or failure of the healing process has a tremendous impact on the patient's quality of life as well as his family's quality of life. Early intervention can mean that a patient with a diabetic foot ulcer can avoid amputation or a paraplegic patient with an ischial ulcer can once again sit up and lead an active life.

Chronic ulcers pose a particularly difficult problem, not only for individual practitioners but also for the healthcare industry as a whole. Treating chronic ulcers is expensive because they're difficult to heal. Consequently, emphasis should be placed on early intervention and prevention.

Winning in wound healing

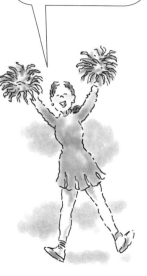

In wound care, you may be able to foresee problems by recognising signs of complications or failure to heal. Give me an H! Give me an E! Give me an A! Give me an L! What does that spell? Heal!

Now that you know what to look for when things aren't going well, let's take a look at what you can expect to see when healing is progressing smoothly. In this case, the patient:
- is well hydrated, well nourished, comfortable and warm
- is well managed for associated or contributing diseases, such as diabetes, heart failure or renal failure
- exhibits normal immune system response.
  In addition, the wound itself:
- receives the oxygen and nutrients it needs (an adequate vascular supply)
- is moist and protected from the environment
- is free from necrotic tissue.
  These conditions optimise wound healing. By using the assessment techniques presented in this chapter, you'll be a part of this success.

Sweet success

Wound healing isn't always straight forward. Through vigilance and consistent assessment and documentation, success is much more likely. By using most of your senses, you can have a tremendous influence on whether a wound heals or becomes chronic and harder to manage. Recognising the signs that warn of failure to heal, and knowing the appropriate interventions, make you a part of the winning wound healing team!

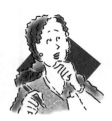

Quick quiz

1. A wound that extends through the epidermis and part way into the dermis is classified as a:
     A.   chronic wound
     B.   acute wound
     C.   partial-thickness wound
     D.   full-thickness wound.

Answer: C. Partial-thickness wounds extend into but not through the dermis, which retains function that helps the healing process.

2. Which wound bed colour indicates normal, healthy granulation tissue?
A. red/pink
B. yellow
C. tan
D. black.

Answer: A. red/pink tissue in a wound bed indicates healthy granulation tissue.

3. If you see multiple colours in a wound bed, you should describe the wound according to the:
A. percentage of tissue types
B. least healthy colour you see
C. colour most visible
D. least percentage of tissue.

Answer: A. Describe a wound with multiple colours according to the percentage of tissue types in the wound bed.

4. Wound healing is facilitated by:
A. a dark environment
B. exposure to air
C. a dry environment
D. a moist environment.

Answer: D. Moisture in the wound bed allows the cells and chemicals needed for healing to move across the wound surface.

5. The PUSH tool is useful for:
A. measuring the size of a pressure ulcer
B. detecting wound infection
C. tracking pressure ulcer healing
D. measuring the depth of a pressure ulcer.

Answer: C. The PUSH tool allows you to track pressure ulcer healing.

6. Which term could be used to accurately describe exudate that's thin and bright red?
A. serous
B. sanguineous
C. serosanguineous
D. purulent.

Answer: B. Sanguineous drainage is red, due to the presence of fresh blood.

7. Which is an appropriate intervention for a wound that has tunnelling?

    A.   provide warmth to the area
    B.   perform conservative sharp debridement
    C.   protect the area from pressure
    D.   no intervention is necessary.

Answer: C. Because tunnelling may be caused by pressure over bony prominences, the wound should be protected.

8. What would your assessment of a non-healing wound show if the cause was a too-dry wound bed?

    A.   rolled skin edges
    B.   maceration
    C.   red, hot skin
    D.   undermining.

Answer: A. A wound bed that's too dry exhibits rolled skin edges and requires moisture-retentive dressings or debridement.

Scoring

 If you answered all eight questions correctly, stand up and bow! You're a wound care all-star.

If you answered five to seven questions correctly, great job! You're a cut above the rest.

If you answered fewer than five questions correctly, don't worry! You've just skinned the surface of wound care; there are nine more chapters to go.

References

Baker, E.A. and Leaper, D.J. (2000) Proteinases, their inhibitors and cytokine profiles in acute wound fluid. *Wound Repair and Regeneration* 8(5):392–398.

Cutting, K.F. (1998) Identification of infection in granulating wounds by registered nurses. *Journal of Clinical Nursing* 7(6):539–546.

Department of Health. (2001) *Good Practice in Consent Implementation Guide: Consent to Examination or Treatment.* London: The Department of Health.

Moffatt, C.J., Franks, P.K. and Hollinworth, H. (2002) Understanding wound pain and trauma: an international perspective. In European Wound Management Association Position Document: Pain at wound dressing changes. London, MEP 2-7.

Robinson, M.K., Trujillo, E.B., Mogensen, K.M. *et al.* (2003) Improving nutritional screening of hospitalised patients – the role of pre-albumin. *Journal of Parental and Enteral Nutrition* 27:389–395.

Sussman, C. and Bates-Jensen, B.M. (2006) *Wound care: A Collaborative Practice Manual.* New York: Lippincott Williams & Wilkins.

Thomas, S. (1997) Assessment and management of wound exudate. *Journal of Wound Care* 6(7):327–330.

Winter, G.D. (1962) Formation of the scab and the rate of epithelialisation of superficial wounds in the young domestic pig. *Nature* 193:293–294.

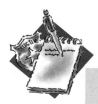

③ Basic wound care procedures

Just the facts

In this chapter, you'll learn:
- ◆ components of a wound care plan
- ◆ wound cleaning and irrigation techniques
- ◆ dressing application techniques
- ◆ debridement techniques
- ◆ specimen collection techniques.

A look at wound care plans

When you have completed the wound assessment you will be ready to write a wound care plan for your patient. A good wound care plan will tell you what the wound related problems are, how each problem should be managed and what the aim of care for each problem is. Wound care plans are usually written by nurses, however, any qualified healthcare professional working with the patient may write or contribute to the care plan. Many organisations have specific policies and procedures in place for different types of wounds, these should be referred to when writing the care plan. The care plan should then be kept in a place where all members of the team caring for the patient can see and refer to it.

What to include

Keep in mind the following list of essential information that you should include in your wound assessment and wound care plan documentation:
- cause of wound, description of wound bed and wound margins, location, size, exudate level

Make sure that your wound care plans contain all the necessary information.

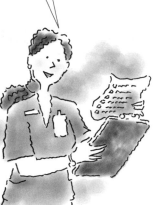

- cleaning agent and method to be used
- type of dressing for the primary and, if needed, secondary layers
- method of securing dressings
- frequency of dressing changes
- time frame for evaluating and changing dressings.

Typically, if there's no change in the wound in 2 weeks, the patient's condition and wound should be reassessed and the care plan should be revised accordingly. If no healing progress is apparent after 2–4 weeks of treatment, referral to a tissue viability nurse (sometimes called a wound care nurse) is recommended. Local policy on when and how to refer to the tissue viability nurse should be followed.

Determining a wound care plan

Wound care is based on the whole patient: his condition, his needs, and the wound profile. The goals of wound care include:
- promoting wound healing by controlling or eliminating causative factors
- preventing or managing infection
- removing non-viable tissue (debridement) as needed
- ensuring adequate blood supply
- providing nutritional and fluid support
- establishing and maintaining a clean, moist, protected wound bed
- managing wound exudate or drainage
- maintaining the skin surrounding the wound to ensure that it remains dry and intact.

For most wounds, promote healing by keeping the wound bed moist, clean and free from debris. However, requirements for providing wound care vary according to the patient assessment and the nature of the wound. (See *Guide to making wound care decisions*, page 63.)

Basic wound care

Basic wound care centres on cleaning and dressing the wound. Before commencing any wound related procedure, ensure the patient understands and agrees with what is going to happen. All procedures carried out should be documented clearly in the nursing record according to the Nursing and Midwifery Council standards (NMC 2007).

Cleaning and dressing the wound are procedures usually carried out using an aseptic technique with particular care taken when the patient is at high risk of developing an infection i.e. is immunocompromised. Sometimes however, it is appropriate to

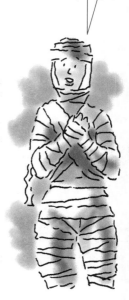

No need to keep it under wraps. Everyone should know that basic wound care involves cleaning and dressing the wound.

Get wise to wounds

Guide to making wound care decisions

Ask yourself the following questions to help you determine what kind of care your patient's wound needs and how you should proceed. Make sure you assess the wound and document according to your organisation's facility's policy and procedure.

How should I clean the wound?
___ Water ___ Saline ___

Is the wound partial-thickness or full-thickness?
___ Partial ___ Full

Is the wound clean, necrotic or infected?
___ Clean ___ Necrotic ___ Infected

Is gangrene present?
___ Yes ___ No

Is there blood flow to the area?
___ Yes ___ No

Does the wound need debridement?
___ Yes ___ No

What kind of debridement is appropriate?
___ Sharp ___ Surgical ___ Biosurgical ___ Autolytic ___ Mechanical

How much drainage is present?
___ None ___ Minimal ___ Moderate ___ Heavy

How does the surrounding skin appear?
___ Intact ___ Irritated ___ Denuded

What dressing is appropriate?
___ Transparent film ___ Hydrogel ___ Hydrocolloid ___ Alginate ___ Foam
___ Hydrofibre ___ Other

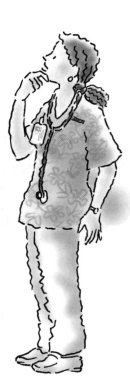

use a clean technique if the wound is likely to be already colonised with bacteria. Traumatic wounds such as gardening or road traffic injuries become contaminated during injury and quickly colonise with bacteria. Wounds such as leg and pressure ulcers, that are often open for long periods of time, also become colonised quickly. The decision to use aseptic or clean technique should be made on the basis of risk of infection to the patient. Individual patient circumstances, the cause of wound and the environment in which they are cared for should all be considered.

Clean machine

The goal of wound cleaning is to remove debris and contaminants from the wound without damaging healthy tissue. The wound should be cleaned initially; repeat cleaning as needed or with each dressing change.

Dress to impress

The basic purpose of a dressing is to provide an optimal environment in which the body can heal itself. Consider this environment before you select a dressing. Functions of a wound dressing include:
- protecting the wound from contamination and trauma
- providing compression if bleeding
- maintaining warmth
- managing moisture levels
- debriding necrotic or sloughy tissue
- filling the wound cavity
- protecting the skin surrounding the wound
- enhancing psychological well-being e.g. pain relief, cosmetic appearance

Follow the golden rule

The cardinal rule is to keep wound tissue moist and surrounding tissue dry. Ideally, a dressing should keep the wound moist, absorb drainage or debris, conform to the wound bed and be adhesive to surrounding skin yet also be easily removable. It should also be user-friendly, require minimal changes, decrease the need for a secondary dressing layer, be cost-effective and both comfortable and aesthetically acceptable to the patient.

What you need

Here is a list of what you will need:
- hypoallergenic tape or elastic netting
- dressings trolley or suitably clean surface if in patient's own home

- 1 × sterile dressing pack
- 50–60 ml syringe-tip syringe
- 2 × pair sterile gloves
- sterile normal saline (0.9%)
- spare gauze (if needed)
- selected topical dressing
- procedure pad
- disposable wound-measuring devices.

Getting ready

Confirm the patient's identity according to your local policy. Then assemble the equipment at the patient's bedside. Use clean or sterile technique as appropriate. If required cut tape into strips for securing dressings. Loosen lids/open seals on cleaning solutions and open dressing packs for easy removal. Attach the disposable clinical waste bag to the trolley (or table) to hold clinical waste.

How you do it

Before any dressing change, wash your hands and follow the principles of standard precautions.

Cleaning the wound

First decide if cleaning is necessary. A healthy wound bed that is healing well may not need cleaning. Remember, cleaning (particularly mechanical cleaning) can damage fragile new tissue.
- Provide privacy and explain the procedure to the patient to allay his fears and promote cooperation.
- Position the patient in a way that maximises his comfort while allowing easy access to the wound site.
- Cover bed linen with a procedure pad to prevent soiling.

Gently does it

- Open the dressing pack and spread out the sterile field, being careful not to contaminate. Open the cleaning solution container and carefully pour cleaning solution into the bowl, avoiding splashing. (See *Choosing a cleaning agent*, page 66.)
- Carefully 'drop' the sterile dressing onto the sterile field without contaminating.
- Put on the first pair of gloves.
- Gently roll or lift an edge of the soiled dressing to obtain a starting point. Support adjacent skin firmly while gently releasing the soiled dressing from the skin. When possible, remove the dressing in the direction of hair growth. Take care not to traumatise

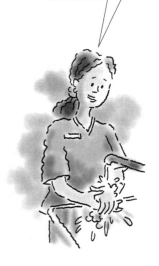

Before any dressing change, be sure to wash your hands. Always follow standard precautions during the procedure.

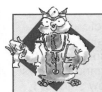

Get wise to wounds

Choosing a cleaning agent

In the UK and the rest of Europe, the most commonly used cleaning agent is sterile normal saline (0.9%). Sterile normal saline (0.9%) is isotonic (it is compatible with body fluids) and non-toxic, and can therefore be used safely on all wound types. It is relatively cheap and contributes to a moist wound healing environment. Patients who are at an increased risk of infection, such as those who are immunocompromised e.g. through disease or drug therapy, should have their wounds cleaned with sterile normal saline (0.9%).

An alternative cleaning solution is potable (drinkable) tap water. Tap water can be used to clean dirty or contaminated wounds such as cuts or grazes and chronic open wounds such as leg ulcers. In A&E departments, for example, when the priority is to clean a traumatic wound of any visible contaminants such as gravel or soil, the wound can be held under a running tap. This will usually remove surface debris effectively. In the community, the patient may clean their chronic wound with tap water prior to the nurse's visit. Chronic wounds are likely to be heavily colonised with bacteria and therefore using tap water to clean them is unlikely to introduce infection.

A review of the research relating to infection rates and the use of tap water and normal saline (0.9%) concluded that there was no evidence that using tap water to cleanse acute wounds in adults increases infection (Fernandez and Griffiths 2008). The review suggested that more research on the subject is needed.

In the past, antiseptic solutions were often used as wound cleaning solutions.
Examples of antiseptic solutions include:

- hydrogen peroxide
- acetic acid
- sodium hypochlorite (Dakin's fluid)
- povidone–iodine.

The strength, volume and contact time are all factors in the effectiveness of any antiseptics. So also is the nature of tissue/debris they come into contact with. Antiseptics are often inactivated in the presence of organic matter such as blood and necrotic tissue. The use of antiseptics has diminished in recent years in recognition of their potential to damage healthy tissue and delay healing (Scanlon and Stubbs 2002) and because of concerns about the development of microbial resistance as a result of their widespread use (McDonnell and Denver Russell 1999).

skin by removing the dressing too quickly. Silicone-based adhesive removers can help to loosen firmly adhered adhesive dressings.
- Inspect the dressing for discoloration and saturation. Ensure the complete dressing is removed.
- Place the soiled dressing and your contaminated gloves in the disposable clinical waste bag to avoid contaminating the sterile field. Then wash your hands.
- Put on a clean pair of gloves.
- Inspect the wound. Note the colour, amount and odour of exudate and necrotic debris.
- Inspect the skin around the wound for redness, heat and moisture.

Wound irrigation

Fragile and healing wounds can be gently irrigated to remove surface debris and excess exudate without damaging the wound bed. Irrigation also helps prevent premature surface healing over an abscess pocket or infected tract:

- Use your syringe to draw up 50–60 ml of normal saline (0.9%), hold syringe at a 45° angle to the wound and point downwards.
- Wearing protective eye goggles and apron, depress plunger slowly to irrigate excess exudate and debris from wound bed.
- Wash your hands.

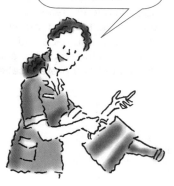

Irrigation cleans tissues and gently flushes away cell debris from an open wound.

Way on down

- Deep cavity wounds can be irrigated more thoroughly using a sterile soft silicone catheter and syringe.
- Don protective eye goggles and apron.
- Fill the syringe with the irrigating solution and connect the catheter to the syringe.
- Gently instill a slow, steady stream of solution into the wound until the syringe empties. (See *Irrigating a deep wound*, page 68.) Where possible make sure the solution flows from the clean to the dirty area of the wound to prevent contamination of clean tissue by exudate. Also make sure the solution reaches all areas of the wound.
- Refill the syringe, reconnect it to the catheter and repeat the irrigation. Continue to irrigate the wound until the solution returns clear. Note the amount of solution administered. Then remove and discard the catheter and syringe in the disposable clinical waste bag. (See *Wound irrigation tips*, page 69.)

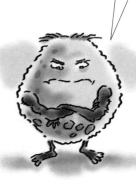

If you aren't careful during irrigation, my pathogenic friends and I will run rampant.

Positioned for success

- Keep the patient positioned to allow further wound drainage into the basin.
- Clean the area around the wound with normal saline (0.9%) and pat dry with gauze; wipe intact surrounding skin with a skin protectant wipe and allow it to dry.
- Apply dressing according to wound care plan.
- Remove and discard your gloves and gown.
- Make sure the patient is comfortable.
- Dispose of all soiled equipment and supplies according to your local infection control policy.

Get wise to wounds

Irrigating a deep wound

When preparing to irrigate a wound, use a 50–60 ml catheter tip syringe, a soft silicone catheter (sterile) and warmed normal saline (0.9%). Explain the procedure, position the patient to aid drainage, then carefully place the catheter into the wound base and hold it there taking care not to exert any pressure or force onto the wound or surrounding tissues. Position an emesis bowl beneath the wound and protect patient and sheets with linen saver.

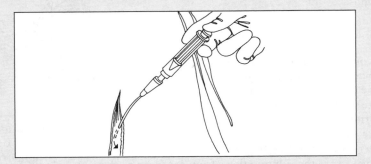

Irrigate the wound with a gentle pressure until you've administered the full amount and the solution returns clear. Keep the emesis bowl under the wound to collect any remaining drainage.

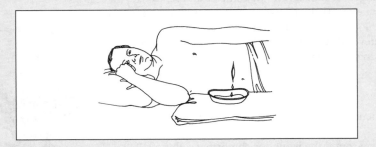

Mechanical cleansing

Occasionally, it is necessary to clean the wound bed mechanically (by wiping rather than irrigation), for example when irrigation fails to remove visible debris/contaminants from the wound bed.

• Dip the sterile gauze pad (folded if necessary) into the normal saline (0.9%) and use to clean wound.

Get wise to wounds

Wound irrigation tips

How can you avoid mess or spillage when irrigating a wound in a hard-to-reach location? Here are some tips you can follow.

Limb wounds

You can soak an arm or a leg wound in a large vessel of fluid such as water or normal saline solution lined with a disposable liner. Remember that this method is contraindicated in patient's with cellulitis and unstable coagulation studies.

If possible, rinse the wound several times and carefully dispose of the contaminated liquid. Reserve the equipment you used for that particular patient. Dry and store it after cleaning it in accordance with your local infection control policy.

Trunk or thigh wounds

Because they're difficult to irrigate, trunk or thigh wounds require some ingenuity. One method uses Stomahesive and a plastic irrigating chamber applied over the wound. (Run warm solution through an infusion set and collect it in a drainage bag.)

You can also use a syringe for irrigation. Where possible, direct the flow at right angles to the wound and allow the fluid to drain by gravity. Doing so requires careful positioning of the patient, either in bed or on a chair. The patient may need analgesia during the treatment.

If irrigation isn't possible, you'll have to swab the wound clean, which is time-consuming. Swab away exudate before using saline solution to clean the wound (taking care not to push loose debris into the wound).

- Where possible wipe gently from the least-contaminated area to the most contaminated area. For a linear-shaped wound, such as an incision, gently wipe from top to bottom in one motion. For an open wound, such as a pressure ulcer, gently wipe in concentric circles, again starting directly over the wound and moving outwards.
- Discard the used gauze pad in the clinical waste bag.
- Using a clean gauze pad for each wiping motion, repeat the procedure until you've cleaned the entire wound (and surrounding skin if needed).

Practice pointers

- Allow the cleaning solution to reach room temperature. If you have access to a warming cabinet (a cabinet designed specifically for warming fluids and often used in theatre or intensive therapy unit (ITU)) warm

it to 37°C. This will be more comfortable for your patient and prevent cooling the wound bed which can lead to delays in healing.
• Never use a needle to irrigate; there is a risk of needle-stick injury to you and your patient.
• Never use a cotton ball or a cotton-filled gauze pad to clean a wound because cotton fibres left in the wound may cause contamination or a foreign body reaction.

Made to measure

• Measure the surface area of the wound with a disposable wound-measuring device, a cm² grid for example. (See Chapter 2, *Get out your ruler*, page 42.) Know your organisation's policy for wound measurement and always be consistent with colleagues in your measurement technique.
• Measure the depth of a full-thickness wound. Gently insert a sterile flexible foam-tipped device into the deepest part of the wound bed and place a mark on the stick where it meets the skin level. Measure the marked device to determine wound depth (although this will not tell you the variable depth of the wound, it will tell you the deepest point of the wound).

Testing for tunnelling

• Gently probe the wound bed and edges with your finger or with a sterile flexible foam-tipped device to assess for wound tunnelling or undermining. Tunnelling usually signals wound extension along fascial planes. Gauge tunnel depth by determining how far you can insert your finger or the foam-tipped device.
• Next, reassess the condition of the skin and wound. Note the character of the cleaned wound bed and the surrounding skin.
• Prepare to apply the appropriate topical dressing. Instructions for applying hydrocolloid, transparent film, alginate, foam and hydrogel dressings follow. (See *Choosing a wound dressing*, page 71.) For other dressings or topical agents, follow the manufacturer's instructions and/or seek advice from your tissue viability nurse.

This tunnel sure is deep! When testing for wound tunnelling, remember to gently probe the wound bed.

Applying a hydrocolloid dressing

Hydrocolloid dressings can be used to rehydrate the wound bed and to promote autolysis.

Choose a pre-sized dressing or cut one to overlap the wound by about 2.5 cm. Remove the dressing from its package, pull the release paper from the adherent side of the dressing, and apply the dressing to the wound. Hold the dressing in place with your hand (the warmth will mould the dressing to the skin).

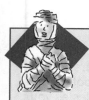

Dress for success

Choosing a wound dressing

The patient's needs and wound characteristics determine which type of dressing you'll use on a wound.

Gauze dressings

Made of absorptive cotton or synthetic fabric, gauze dressings are permeable to water, water vapour and oxygen, and may be impregnated with a hydrogel or other agent. Gauze has a tendency to stick to the wound bed, causing wound bed trauma and pain on removal. It can also result in wound bed cooling due to its loose, open weave which allows heat from the wound to pass straight through. For these reasons it is not suitable as a permanent wound dressing although it may be moistened with saline solution and used as a temporary measure in an emergency.

Hydrocolloid dressings

Hydrocolloid dressings are adhesive, mouldable wafers made of a carbohydrate-based material that usually have waterproof backings. They're impermeable to oxygen, water and water vapour, and most have some absorptive properties. They rehydrate the wound and promote autolysis and healing.

Transparent film dressings

Transparent film dressings are clear, adherent and non-absorptive. These polymer-based dressings are permeable to oxygen and water vapour but not to water. Their transparency allows visual inspection. Because they can't absorb drainage, they're used on partial-thickness wounds with minimal exudate.

Hydrofibre dressings

Hydrofibre dressings are soft, white dressings available as flat dressings or ropes. They are made primarily from a carbohydrate-based material (carboxymethylcellulose) which is very absorptive. Hydrofibres can be used on infected wounds. They maintain their integrity well even in very moist conditions and they are usually easy to remove from the wound. They promote autolysis and healing but should be discontinued as exudate diminishes.

Alginate dressings

Made from seaweed, alginate dressings are non-woven, absorptive dressings available as soft sterile pads or ropes. They absorb excessive exudate and may be used on infected wounds. As these dressings absorb exudate, they turn into a gel that keeps the wound bed moist and promotes healing. When exudate is no longer excessive, switch to another type of dressing.

Foam dressings

Foam dressings are conformable, sponge-like polymer dressings that may be impregnated or coated with other materials. These are absorptive dressings that may or may not have an adhesive backing. These dressings promote moist wound healing and are useful when a non-adherent surface is desired.

Hydrogel dressings

Water-based and non-adherent, hydrogel dressings are polymer-based dressings that have some (limited) absorptive properties. They're used when the wound needs moisture. Available as a gel in a tube, as flexible sheets and as saturated gauze strips; some have a specific cooling effect.

Smooth operator

• As you apply the dressing, carefully smooth out wrinkles and avoid stretching the dressing.
• If the dressing's edges need to be secured with tape, apply a skin sealant (a silicone-based non-sting barrier spray for example) to the intact skin around the wound. After the area dries, tape the dressing to the skin. The sealant protects the skin from tape burns and skin stripping and promotes tape adherence. Avoid using tension or pressure when you apply the tape.
• Remove your gloves and discard them in the disposable clinical waste bag. Dispose of bag according to your infection control policy and then wash your hands.
• Hydrocolloid dressings are usually changed every 3 to 7 days but always check the manufacturer's instructions as products do differ; change it immediately if the patient complains of pain, the dressing no longer adheres or leakage occurs.

Hydrocolloid dressings often have a mild but distinct odour of their own, make sure your patient is aware of this to minimise any worry on their part.

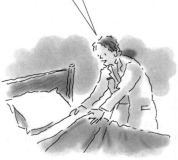

Carefully smooth out wrinkles as you apply the dressing to minimise irritation.

Applying a transparent film dressing

Film dressings can be used to protect the wound bed and retain moisture at the wound interface:
• Select a dressing to overlap the wound by 2.5 to 5 cm.
• Gently lay the dressing over the wound; avoid wrinkling the dressing. To prevent shearing force, don't stretch the dressing over the wound. Press firmly on the edges of the dressing to promote adherence.
• Change the dressing every 3–4 days, depending on the amount of exudate drainage (film dressings are only suitable for low amounts of exudate). If the seal is no longer secure or if accumulated tissue fluid extends beyond the edges of the wound and onto the surrounding skin, change to an absorbent type of dressing.
• When removing, carefully lift a corner of the film and pull forwards in the direction of hair growth, holding the skin down firmly but gently with the other hand. Relax tension on dressing. Resume tension until dressing is completely removed.
• Check manufacturer's instructions for individual product information.

Applying a hydrofibre dressing

• Hydrofibre dressings can be used to absorb excess exudate and promote autolysis.
• Hydrofibres dressings come in flat and rope-type presentations for filling cavities.

- Apply the dressing to the wound surface or lay into the wound cavity (fill the cavity but do not pack). Packing can cause wound pain and necrosis and impedes the dressing's ability to absorb exudate to its full potential.
- Cover with a secondary dressing such as an adhesive foam or hydrocolloid.
- Change the dressing every 3–4 days depending on the exudate levels. Dressings can be left for up to 7 days if exudate levels allow.
- When the exudate diminishes, change to a different dressing.
- Check manufacturer's instructions for individual product information.

Applying an alginate dressing

- Alginate dressings can be used to absorb excess exudate and promote autolysis.
- Like hydrofibres, alginate dressings come in flat and rope-type presentations.
- Apply the dressing to the wound surface or lay into the cavity (do not pack).
- Cover the area with a secondary dressing (such as an adhesive-backed foam dressing).
- If the wound is exuding heavily, change the dressing once or twice daily until drainage decreases, then change the dressing less frequently – every 3 to 4 days. When the exudate diminishes or the wound bed looks dry, stop using the alginate dressing.
- Check manufacturer's instructions for individual product information.

Applying a foam dressing

- Foam dressings can be used to maintain warmth, absorb exudate and protect the wound bed.
- Gently lay the dressing over the wound.
- If non-adhesive, use tape or elastic netting to hold the dressing in place.
- Change the dressing every 3–4 days, when the foam can no longer absorb the exudate.
- Check manufacturer's instructions for individual product information.

Applying a hydrogel dressing

- Hydrogel dressings can be used to rehydrate a dry wound bed and promote autolysis in the presence of slough.
- Apply a moderate amount of gel to the wound bed.

- Cover the area with a secondary dressing (transparent film or foam depending on the exudate level).
- Change the dressing every 2–3 days or as needed to keep the wound bed moist.
- Hydrogel dressings also come as a pre-packaged, saturated gauze for wounds with cavities that require filling 'dead space'. Follow the manufacturer's directions to apply these and any other types of hydrogel dressings.

Other dressings

There are many dressings on the market. If you are using a dressing for the first time make sure you know the correct way to apply and remove it. Read the instruction leaflet and ask for a demonstration if necessary.

Practice pointers

All dressings should be used in accordance with the manufacturer's instructions. Be observant for infection; it may cause foul-smelling exudate, persistent pain, severe erythema, induration and elevated skin and body temperatures. Remember though, some dressings and topical agents may also cause odour. Severe erythema may signal worsening cellulitis, which means the offending organisms have invaded the tissue and are no longer localised. Advancing infection or cellulitis can lead to septicemia and even death and therefore should be reported immediately.

Debridement

Debridement of non-viable tissue is the most important factor in wound management. Wound healing can't take place until non-viable tissue is removed. Non-viable tissue may present as moist yellow or grey tissue (slough) that's separating from viable tissue. Non-viable, necrotic tissue typically presents as thick, hard, leathery black eschar. Areas of necrotic tissue may mask underlying fluid collections or abscesses. Although debridement can be uncomfortable (especially with burns), it's necessary to prevent infection and promote healing.

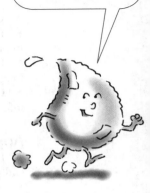

In autolytic debridement, moisture-retentive dressings are placed over the wound and necrotic tissue dissolves in the wound fluid.

Types of debridement

Debridement of necrotic tissue may be accomplished by surgical, sharp, biosurgical, autolytic, enzyme or mechanical techniques.

Surgical debridement

Surgical debridement involves removing both necrotic and healthy tissue from the wound bed with a cutting tool. This procedure converts a chronic wound to a clean, acute wound. It's performed by a surgeon in theatre with the patient under anaesthesia. Caution should be used when performing surgical debridement on patients who have low platelet counts or who are taking anticoagulants.

Conservative sharp debridement

Conservative sharp debridement is the removal of necrotic (non-viable tissue) by scalpel or scissors. Due to the possibility of infection and of trauma to underlying structures this procedure must only be carried out by a *qualified healthcare professional who has received appopriate education and training in sharp debridement techniques.* During conservative sharp debridement, loosened eschar is carefully held with forceps and separated from the viable tissue beneath with a sterile scalpel or pair of scissors. Sharp debridement should be carried out in a clinical procedures (treatment) room to minimise the risk of cross-infection and to ensure the patient's privacy and dignity are maintained. The patient must be given an appropriate analgesia and local pain relief i.e. local anaesthetic, as this procedure can be uncomfortable. If the patient experiences pain, the procedure should be stopped immediately.

Biosurgical debridement

Biosurgical debridement is the removal of soft necrotic or sloughy tissue by larval (maggot) therapy. This involves the use of sterile maggots (from the *Lucilia sericata* fly) which are applied to the wound either in a mesh bag or under a mesh dressing. Specialist dressings and advice on the application procedure are provided by the larval therapy suppliers. The larvae excrete enzymes which dissolve the non-viable tissue; this is then ingested as a source of nutrition. Although some patients (and healthcare professionals) may feel squeamish about using larval therapy, it is an effective form of debridement with fewer risks involved than with surgical or sharp debridement techniques. It is important, however, that your patient fully understands what this therapy involves before you proceed. Check your local policy about the need for informed consent for larval therapy.

Autolytic debridement

Autolytic debridement involves the use of moisture-retentive dressings to cover the wound bed. Necrotic tissue is then softened by enzymes in the wound fluid. Although autolytic debridement takes longer than other debridement methods, it isn't painful, it's easy to do, and it's appropriate for patients who can't tolerate any other method or who are not fit for an anaesthetic. Many dressings promote autolysis including hydrocolloids and hydrogels in dry or low exudate wounds and hydrofibres and alginates for moderate-to-heavily exuding wounds.

Autolytic debridement should not be used if the wound is infected unless suitable systemic antiobiotic therapy is in place.

Enzyme debridement

Debridement with enzymatic agents is a selective method of debridement no longer in use in the UK. Enzyme debridement is expensive and difficult to use, and has not been proven to be any more effective than other conservative methods. The only enzyme debriding agent available in the UK (Varidase®) was discontinued in 2006.

Mechanical debridement

Mechanical debridement methods include surgical and conservative sharp debridement (see above), plus hydrosurgery, pulsatile lavage and hydrotherapy. These latter two methods are rarely used, usually in specialist centres such as burns units.

Hydrosurgery

This new surgical technique involves the use of saline forced under high pressure through a jet nozzle to produce a high velocity stream and create a vacuum. The tool can remove selected pieces of necrotic tissue very quickly, it will also clean the wound and remove surface contaminants. There is, however, a risk of pain and bleeding, and specialist training for use is required.

Finger on the pulse

Pulsatile lavage involves the use of a pressurised antiseptic solution, which cleans tissue and removes wound debris and excess drainage. It is rarely used in the UK.

Whirlpool wizard

Hydrotherapy – commonly referred to as 'tubbing', 'tanking' or 'whirlpool' – involves

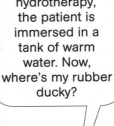

In hydrotherapy, the patient is immersed in a tank of warm water. Now, where's my rubber ducky?

immersing the patient in a tank of warm water, with intermittent agitation of the water. It's usually performed on large wounds with a significant amount of non-viable tissue covering the wound surface (such as burns) but is rarely used in the UK.

Wound specimen collection

Wound specimen collection involves using a sterile alginate-tipped swab, aspiration with a syringe or punch tissue biopsy to help identify pathogens.

Because most wounds are colonised with surface bacteria, the swab specimen technique is limited in that it only obtains surface cultures. Needle aspiration of fluid or punch tissue biopsy is recommended for accurate wound culturing. These procedures must be performed by qualified healthcare professionals with the appropriate training.

What you need

- clean and sterile gloves
- 1 × sterile dressing pack
- normal saline (0.9%)
- sterile wound swab
- sterile culture tube with transport medium
- fresh sterile dressings for the wound
- laboratory request form
- patient labels.

How you do it

- Confirm the patient's identity using two patient identifiers according to your organisation's policy.
- Provide privacy and explain the procedure to the patient.
- Wash your hands, prepare a sterile field and put on clean or sterile gloves.
- Remove the dressing to expose the wound. Dispose of the soiled dressings properly.
- Put on a new pair of gloves.
- Clean the wound with normal saline (0.9%).
- Inspect the wound, noting the colour, amount and odour of exudate and the presence of necrotic debris.

- Gently compress the wound bed to elicit new exudate.
- Using a zig-zag motion, wipe the sterile alginate-tipped swab across the base of the wound bed. Remember, never collect exudate from the skin and then insert the same swab into the wound; this could contaminate the wound with skin bacteria.
- Remove the swab from the wound and immediately place it in the swab culture tube.
- Label the culture tube and send the tube to the laboratory immediately with a completed laboratory request form. Remember to note any antibiotic therapy on the request form and include the wound history and any other relevant factors, e.g. traumatic injury contaminated by garden soil.
- Redress the wound according to the wound care plan.

Practice pointers

If zig-zagging the swab in the wound doesn't provide a specimen, try using a rotating motion over the entire wound bed.

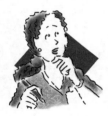

Quick quiz

1. Because sharp debridement may cause trauma to underlying structures, the procedure should only be carried out by:
    A. a healthcare professional
    B. a healthcare assistant
    C. a doctor
    D. a qualified healthcare professional with appropriate education and training.

Answer: D. Sharp debridement carries some risk to the patient and should only be carried out by a healthcare professional with the appropriate education and training.

2. To irrigate a wound, direct the flow of irrigant:
    A. towards the wound
    B. away from the wound
    C. towards the centre of the wound
    D. to pool inside of the wound.

Answer: B. Direct the flow away from the wound to prevent contamination.

3. The most commonly used cleaning agent is:
   A. sterile normal saline (0.9%)
   B. hydrogen peroxide
   C. povidone–iodine solution
   D. sodium hypochlorite.

Answer: A. Sterile normal saline (0.9%) is most commonly used because it provides a moist environment, promotes granulation tissue formation and causes minimal fluid shifts in healthy adults.

4. Wounds should be mechanically cleaned with moistened gauze:
   A. at every dressing change
   B. once a week
   C. only if there is obvious debris in the wound bed
   D. if the wound bed is clean and healing.

Answer: C. Only if there is obvious debris to remove such as loose slough and dressing remnants.

5. Which type of dressing wouldn't be appropriate for a wound with excessive drainage?
   A. foam dressing
   B. transparent film dressing
   C. alginate dressing
   D. hydrofibre dressing.

Answer: B. Because a transparent film dressing can't absorb drainage, it should be used only for wounds with minimal drainage.

6. Which methods of wound culturing are most accurate for determining infection?
   A. swab technique and needle aspiration
   B. swab technique and punch tissue biopsy
   C. aspiration and punch tissue biopsy
   D. aerobic and anaerobic swab techniques.

Answer: C. Because the surface of most wounds are normally colonised with bacteria, swab cultures may not be accurate. Aspiration and punch tissue biopsy provide the most reliable information.

Scoring

✩✩✩ If you answered all six questions correctly, yippee! You're quite a fine specimen.

✩✩ If you answered five questions correctly, great job! You really cleaned up in the area of basic wound care procedures.

✩ If you answered fewer than five questions correctly, don't despair! Review the chapter and try again, you'll clean up in no time.

References

Fernandez, R. and Griffiths, R. (2008) Water for wound cleansing. *Cochrane Database of Systematic Reviews* 2008, Issue 1.

McDonnell, G. and Denver Russell, A. (1999) Antispetics and disinfectants: activity, action and resistance. *Clinical Microbiology Reviews* 12(1):147–179.

Nursing and Midwifery Council (NMC). (2007) *Record Keeping*. London: NMC.

Scanlon, E. and Stubbs, N. (2002) To use or not to use? The debate on the use of antispetics in wound care. *British Journal of Community Nursing (WoundCare)* 7(9)Suppl.: 8–20.

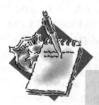

④ Wound care products

Just the facts

In this chapter, you'll learn:

♦ criteria to use when selecting wound care products

♦ types of dressings used in wound care and the characteristics, indications, advantages and disadvantages of each type

♦ products that are used in conjunction with dressings, including their indications, advantages and disadvantages.

A look at wound care products

Over time, wound care has developed from a practice that focused primarily on care of the injury to a process that also considers the complexities of the patient's general health, possible underlying disease and specific wound characteristics. As wound care knowledge has increased, so have the number and types of products available to aid healing.

As you read, keep in mind that wound care products are tools that can help promote full healing, but they aren't the only tools you'll need. Unless concurrent problems, such as malnutrition, circulatory disorders and patient knowledge deficits, are also addressed, the healing process stalls. In addition, no dressing or topical agent can compensate for an incomplete assessment. In short, let the findings of a thorough assessment guide your wound care product selection. (See *Tips for selecting wound care products*, page 82.)

All the rage

Keep in mind that new products arrive almost daily and others are updated or improved regularly. Because the quality of the care that you provide depends on your level of knowledge, it's

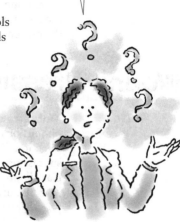

The abundance of commercially prepared dressings and adjunct products – and the fact that many have similar names and functions – can make choosing the right product a daunting task.

Tips for selecting wound care products

When selecting wound care products, let the big picture guide your choices. Ask yourself these important questions:

- Which companies have contracts to supply wound care products to your setting? (Learn about these products first.)
- What's the simplest method of covering the wound? Which is the most cost-effective?
- Are the dressings available on FP10? Is the patient entitled to FP10? If not, can the patient afford the supplies he needs? (Simple and affordable aren't necessarily synonymous.) If not, is financial assistance available?
- Who provides wound care at home? If the patient can't perform this important task, can family members or friends help? Can the community nursing team or the practice nurse provide the required help?
- What caused the wound and how can the cause best be alleviated? (This is especially important when treating chronic wounds; less so when treating acute wounds.)

- How often does the dressing need to be changed? (It usually takes at least 8 hours for a wound to achieve homeostasis after a dressing change. Therefore, the less often dressing changes are needed, the better.)
- How much exudate is present?
- Does the wound need more moisture?
- Should the wound be debrided? If so, which method is best for the patient?
- After cleaning and drying, does the wound (not the dressing) have an unpleasant odour? Do you suspect infection? If so, is a culture warranted?
- Is there tunnelling, undermining or a cavity that needs to be filled?
- Are the wound edges open or closed? (Wound edges must be open for complete healing to occur.)
- How large is the wound? Would it be more cost-effective to use an advanced wound care therapy to facilitate granulation tissue or closure?

imperative that you stay up-to-date by periodically reviewing the available products. It is also important to read the manufacturer's instructions as to when and how to use each dressing so that it is used to optimum benefit for the patient. If in doubt about which dressing to use and how to use it, a tissue viability nurse (a nurse who specialises in the prevention and management of wounds) will be able to advise you.

Wound dressings

Moisture level, tissue adherence, infection control and wound dimensions are just some of the factors that affect wound dressing selection. The level of moisture in the wound bed is critical to the success or failure of healing. Consequently, one fundamental way to classify dressings is by their effect on wound moisture. Ask yourself, does the dressing add, absorb or not affect wound moisture? (See *Dressing for the occasion*, page 83.)

Dressing for the occasion

Some dressings absorb moisture from a wound bed; some add moisture to it. Others help maintain the existing moisture level. Use this chart to quickly determine the category of dressing that's appropriate for your patient.

MOISTURE SCALE

Absorb moisture	Neutral (maintain existing moisture level)	Add moisture
• Alginates • Hydrofibres • Specialty absorptives • Topical negative pressure (TNP) devices	• Foams • Hydrocolloids • Compression bandages	• Composites • TNP devices • Thin foams • Thin hydrocolloids • Honey	• Transparent films • Biological dressings • Collagen dressings • Contact layers	• Sheet hydrogels	• Amorphous hydrogels • Debriding agents

Out with the old

In the past, gauze was a core wound dressing. However, as medical research has afforded an improved understanding of wounds and the healing process, manufacturers have developed new materials and sophisticated dressing options that promote far better healing and patient comfort than gauze ever did.

Modern wound products include alginate, antimicrobial, biological, collagen, composite, contact layer, foam, hydrocolloid, hydrogel, specialty absorptive, silicone and transparent film dressings. Wound fillers are also available.

Alginate dressings

Made from seaweed, alginate dressings are non-woven and absorptive. They're available as soft, sterile pads or ropes. Alginate dressings absorb excessive exudate and may be used on infected wounds. As they absorb exudate, they turn into a gel that keeps the wound bed moist and promotes healing. These non-adhesive and non-occlusive dressings also promote autolysis.

Examples of alginate dressings include:
- Algisite M®
- Kaltostat®
- Sorbsan®.

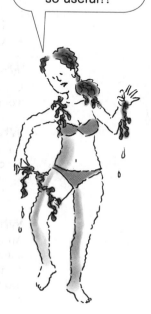

Alginate dressings are made from seaweed. Who knew this stuff was so useful?!

When they're used

Use alginate dressings on wounds with moderate-to-heavy drainage and wounds with undermining.

What's the advantage?

Alginate dressings are beneficial because they:
- may be layered for more absorption
- come in ropes for filling cavity wounds.

What to consider

Irrigation may be needed to remove an alginate dressing from the wound. In addition, alginate dressings:
- require secondary dressings
- can't be used on dry eschar or wounds with light drainage
- may dehydrate the wound bed of a dryer wound.

Antimicrobial dressings

Antimicrobial dressings inhibit or kill bacteria and provide a moist environment for wound healing – an improvement on topical antibiotic therapy. Active ingredients, such as silver, honey and iodine, provide the antimicrobial effects. These dressings come in many forms, including transparent dressings, gauze, island dressings, foams and absorptive fillers.
   Examples of antimicrobial dressings include:
- Acticoat®
- Iodosorb®
- Contreet®

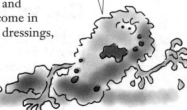

Drats! When a patient has an antimicrobial dressing in place, I don't stand a chance!

When they're used

Use antimicrobial dressings as primary or secondary dressings on wounds that are infected, draining or non-healing.

What's the advantage?

Antimicrobial dressings:
- control bacteria
- work against a variety of different microorganisms
- help control odour and exudate.

What to consider

Antimicrobial dressings may still require the patient to have systemic antibiotic therapy. In addition, antimicrobial dressings may:
- produce a hypersensitivity reaction in patients sensitive to such product ingredients as silver or iodine
- sting when applied

- contribute to the development of resistant organisms (not yet known)
- emit their own chemical odours.

Biological dressings

Biological dressings are temporary dressings that function like skin grafts. They may be made from amnionic or chorionic membranes, woven from manmade fibres or harvested from animals (usually pigs) or cadavers. Eventually, the body will reject a biological dressing. If rejection occurs before the underlying wound heals, the dressing may be replaced with a skin graft.

Examples of biological dressings include:
- Hyalofil-R®, Hyalofil-F®
- Dermagraft® (limited use in the UK).

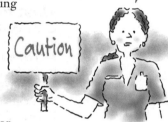

Biological dressings may help your patient's wound heal more quickly but beware of allergic reactions.

Caution

When they're used
Use biological dressings as temporary dressings for ulcers of varying thickness (depending on the product), skin grafting donor sites and burns.

What's the advantage?
The biggest advantage of biological dressings is that they can shorten healing times. They can also:
- prevent infection and fluid loss
- ease patient discomfort.

What to consider
Biological dressings:
- are relatively expensive
- may cause allergic reactions
- usually require secondary dressings
- may require additional training to apply.

Collagen dressings

Collagen dressings, which are usually made from bovine or avian collagen, accelerate wound healing by encouraging the organisation of new collagen fibres and granulation tissue. They're available in gel, granule and sheet forms. Some also contain alginate. Collagen dressings are rarely used in the UK.

Examples of collagen dressings include:
- FIBRACOL PLUS® Collagen Wound Dressing with Alginate
- Medifil® Pads.

When they're used
Use collagen dressings on chronic, non-healing, granulated wound beds and wounds with tunnelling.

What's the advantage?
Collagen dressings:
- are effective on chronic, clean wounds
- can be used on wounds with minimal-to-heavy drainage (depending on the product selected)
- are easy to apply.

What to consider
Collagen dressings aren't appropriate for third-degree burns or wounds with dry beds. In addition, they may:
- cause an allergic reaction if the patient is sensitive to collagen, bovine or avian products
- require secondary dressings.

Remember, patients should be informed that the dressing is derived in part from animals as they may express ethical or religious objections to using them.

Collagen dressings are made from bovine or avian collagen. Remember that these dressings can cause an allergic reaction in patients sensitive to bovine or avian products.

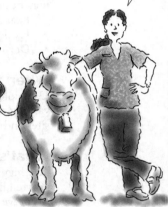

Composite dressings

Composite dressings are hybrid dressings that combine two or more types of dressings into one. For example, a three-layer composite dressing can include a bacterial barrier; an absorbent foam, hydrocolloid or hydrogel layer; an adherent or a non-adherent layer; and an adhesive border.

Examples of composite dressings include:
- Combiderm®
- TELFA Plus® Island Dressing.

When they're used
Use composite dressing on wounds with minimal-to-heavy drainage.

What's the advantage?
Composite dressings are:
- all-in-one dressings that come in various combinations to suit each patient's wound care needs
- available in multiple sizes and shapes.

What to consider
Composite dressings can't be used on third-degree burns. In addition, they:
- may dry the wound bed if very absorbent
- can't be cut to fit without losing some of the dressing's integrity.

Contact layer dressings

Contact layer dressings are single-layer dressings made of woven or perforated material suitable for direct contact with the wound's surface. The low-adherent contact layer prevents other dressings from sticking to the surface of the wound.

Examples of contact layer dressings include:
* Mepitel®
* Urgotul®
* N/A Ultra®.

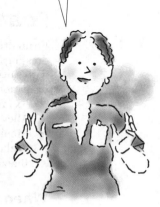

What a relief! Contact layer dressings decrease the pain experienced by the patient during dressing changes.

When they're used
Use contact layer dressings to let drainage flow to a secondary dressing while preventing that dressing from adhering to the wound.

What's the advantage?
Contact layer dressings:
* decrease the pain experienced during dressing changes
* can be cut to fit or overlap the wound edges
* can be cost-effective when used in combination with a cheaper absorbent secondary dressing.

What to consider
Contact layer dressings require a secondary dressing and are contraindicated for use on third-degree burns, infected wounds and wounds with tunnelling.

Enzyme-based debriding agents

When applied directly to necrotic or devitalised tissue, enzyme-based debriding agents remove dead tissue in a wound. An example of a debriding agent is Varidase®.

When they're used
Enzyme-based debriding agents are intended for use on wounds with moderate amounts of dry necrotic tissue, especially in cases where surgical debridement isn't an option.

What's the advantage?
There is no evidence to suggest enzyme-based debriding agents are more effective than other products.

What to consider.

Debriding agents are expensive. In addition, they may:
* contain known allergens
* require secondary dressings

- be difficult to prepare
- cause irritation if they come in contact with surrounding skin
- cause a burning sensation in the wound during application that can last for several hours.

In Europe, the use of enzyme-based debriding agents has declined in recent years due to a lack of evidence supporting their continued use. In the UK specifically, Varidase® was discontinued in 2006.

Foam dressings

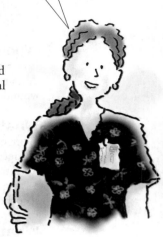

Use a foam dressing on a wound with minimal-to-moderate drainage when you need a nonadherent surface.

Foam dressings are low-adherent, absorbent sponge-like polymer dressings that may include an adhesive border; some are impregnated with silicone. They provide a moist healing environment and thermal insulation; some are impregnated with silicone.

Examples of foam dressings include:
- Allevyn® (flat and cavity)
- Mepilex®
- Tielle Plus®
- Biatain®.

When they're used

Use foam dressings as primary or secondary dressings on wounds with minimal-to-moderate drainage (including around tubes) when you need a low-adherent surface.

What's the advantage?

Foam dressings may be used in combination with other products such as alginates and hydrofibres, and those with an adhesive border don't require a secondary dressing. In addition, foam dressings:
- can be used on infected wounds if changed daily
- can manage heavier drainage because they wick moisture from the wound and allow evaporation (hydropolymer foam dressings)
- can be used around tubes (such as a tracheostomy) because they don't fray like gauze
- conform to difficult-to-dress areas
- are comfortable for the patient.

What to consider

Without an adhesive border, foam dressings may require a secondary dressing, tape, bandage or net. In addition, they:
- may stick to the wound bed if it is dry
- can't manage large amounts of drainage on their own
- may cause maceration if not changed regularly

Honey dressings

Products containing honey are available in a number of different presentations including gel, ointment, adhesive bordered and mesh.

Examples of honey dressings include:

- Mesitran®
- Medihoney®.

When they are used

Use honey dressings as primary dressings when the wound requires desloughing or odour control.

What's the advantage?

Honey dressings are beneficial because they:

- maintain a moist wound environment
- control malodour
- can be used on a variety of wounds
- can be effective on infected wounds (depends on product used).

What to consider

Many honey products require secondary dressings. In addition, they:

- are not suitable for heavily exuding wounds
- are not suitable for full-thickness burns or deep, narrow cavities
- are not always suitable for infected wounds (some products have antimicrobial properties, some do not; always check the product information before using).

Hydrocolloid dressings

Hydrocolloid dressings are adhesive, mouldable wafers made of a carbohydrate-based material. Most have a waterproof backing. They're impermeable to oxygen, water and water vapour, and most provide some degree of absorption. These dressings turn to gel as they absorb moisture, help maintain a moist wound bed and promote autolytic debridement.

Examples of hydrocolloid dressings include:

- DuoDERM®; Granuflex®
- Tegaderm™
- Comfeel®.

When they're used

Use hydrocolloid dressings on wounds with minimal-to-moderate drainage, including wounds with necrosis or slough. Hydrocolloid sheet dressings can also serve as secondary dressings.

What's the advantage?

Hydrocolloid dressings are beneficial because they:

- are low-adherent and moisture retentive
- maintain moisture by becoming gelatinous as they absorb drainage
- may require changing only one to two times each week
- can be easily removed from the wound base
- are available in contoured forms for use on specific sites
- are available in several varieties (sheets, filler or gel) and in thin and traditional thickness.

What to consider

Hydrocolloid dressings:

- may have an odour when removed (some makes only)
- can cause skin stripping when removed incorrectly
- should not be used on fragile skin
- can cause maceration or hypergranulation
- may need to be held in place to maximise adhesion
- should not be used on sensitive skin.

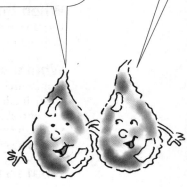

Did you know that hydrocolloid dressings turn to gel as they absorb drainage, which helps promote a moist wound bed?

Aww . . . I just love moisture!

Hydrogel dressings

Hydrogel dressings are water- or glycerin-based polymer dressings that don't adhere to wounds. They provide limited absorption (some are 96% water themselves) and are available as tubes of gel or in flexible sheets. Hydrogel dressings add moisture and promote autolytic debridement.

Examples of hydrogel dressings include:

- Aquasorb®
- Intrasite®
- Granugel®.

When they're used

Use hydrogel dressings on dry wounds, wounds with minimal drainage or wounds with necrosis or slough.

What's the advantage?

Hydrogel dressings come in sheet and amorphous gel form. Some are specifically designed to cool and sooth painful wounds e.g. ActiFormCool®.

What to consider

Hydrogel dressings in gel form require a secondary dressing. In addition, they:

- can macerate surrounding skin if overused

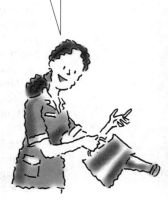

Using a hydrogel dressing is like watering a flower bed. The dressing provides moisture to the wound bed.

- may necessitate daily dressing changes
- vary in viscosity among brands and according to the product's base (water or glycerin).

Hydrofibre dressings (protease modulating)

Hydrofibre dressings are made from sodium carboxymethylcellulose and contain hollow fibres which allow maximum absorption of wound exudate. They maintain a moist environment for healing, promote autolysis and lift skin damaging proteases away from the wound bed.

Example of hydrofibre dressing:
- Aquacel®.

When they're used

Use hydrofibre dressings on infected or non-infected wounds with moderate-to-heavy drainage.

What's the advantage?

Hydrofibre dressings
- are highly absorbent
- are available in a variety of forms
- hold together well even when wet
- minimise wound bed trauma on removal
- reduce wound pain associated with dressing changes.

What to consider

Hydrofibres can't be used on wounds with dry necrosis or with little or no drainage.

Silicone dressings

Silicone dressings are either made of or coated with soft silicone, an inert polymer which minimises tissue adherence and so reduces wound bed trauma and pain on removal. Silicone dressings come in a variety of formulations such as wound contact layers, absorbent foams and skin tapes.

Examples of silicone dressings include:
- Mepitel®
- N/A Ultra®.

When they're used

Use silicone dressings when the wound bed is fragile and when the wound is painful (particularly at dressing change). Silicone dressings are best for clean wounds with a low-to-moderate amount of exudate.

What's the advantage?

Silicone dressings:

- reduce wound pain
- minimise damage to the wound bed
- can be used on fragile, easily torn skin
- some can be used under compression bandages.

What to consider

Silicone dressings can be expensive and some can be difficult to handle. They may also require a secondary dressing/bandage to absorb wound exudate and hold them *in situ*.

Transparent film dressings

Transparent film dressings are clear, adherent, non-absorptive, polyurethane dressings. They're semi-permeable to oxygen and water vapour but not to water itself. Transparency allows visual inspection of the wound while the dressing is in place. Transparent film dressings maintain a moist wound environment.

Examples of transparent film dressings include:

- Bioclusive®
- OpSite Flexigrid®
- Tegaderm®.

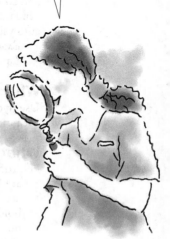

Transparent film dressings allow for visual inspection of the wound while the dressing is in place.

When they're used

Use transparent film dressings on partial-thickness wounds with minimal exudate and as secondary dressings for enhanced moisture retention.

What's the advantage?

Transparent film dressings:

- may require fewer changes
- allow you to see the wound without removing the dressing
- are adherent but won't stick to the wound
- aren't bulky.

What to consider

Transparent film dressings don't absorb drainage, making them appropriate only for shallow partial-thickness wounds with minimal exudate. In addition, the adhesive border can strip skin around the wound when the dressing is removed.

Wound fillers

Wound fillers are specialised dressings used to fill cavity wounds. They're made of various materials and come in many forms, including pastes, granules and foams. Wound fillers can add moisture to the wound bed or absorb drainage, depending on the product.

Examples of wound filler include:

- Allevyn cavity®
- Cavi Care®.

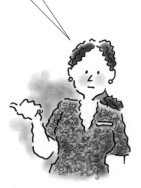

Remember, some wound fillers add moisture to the wound bed while others absorb drainage.

When they're used

Use wound fillers as primary dressings in cavities with minimal-to-moderate drainage that require filling.

What's the advantage?

Wound fillers come in several forms with different absorption abilities.

What to consider

Wound fillers require secondary dressings to secure them into place.

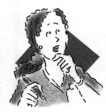

Quick quiz

1. What type of dressing is most appropriate for a patient with a dry wound?

    A. absorptive
    B. hydrogel
    C. alginate
    D. foam.

Answer: B. A dry wound needs added moisture to promote wound healing, so a hydrogel dressing should be used.

2. Which dressing type is most absorbent?

    A. hydrocolloid
    B. foam
    C. hydrogel
    D. hydrofibre.

Answer: D. Although all of these products have some absorptive capacity, hydrofibre dressings are the most absorbent.

3. What's the advantage of using a low-adherent wound contact layer?

    A. It can reduce dressings costs.
    B. It can minimise wound bed trauma on removal.
    C. It can reduce pain at dressing change.
    D. It can reduce frequency of primary dressing changes.

Answer: A, B, C and D. A wound contact layer can do all of the above.

4. You smell an unpleasant odour as you remove your patient's dressing. Which type of dressing may cause this?
  A. alginate
  B. hydrocolloid
  C. composite
  D. foam.

Answer: B. Hydrocolloid dressings absorb drainage and turn to gel. Some (not all) hydrocolloid gels have a distinctive smell.

5. Your patient has a fragile, painful wound which has a low amount of exudate and a clean wound bed. Which of the following dressings would be most suitable?
  A. silicone
  B. hydrofibre
  C. alginate
  D. enzyme-based debriding agent

Answer: A. Silicone is kind to the skin and reduces pain on dressing removal.

Scoring

 If you answered all five questions correctly, shout it out! Your knowledge of wound care products is second to none.

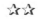 If you answered four questions correctly, well done! You've obviously absorbed all the material on wound care products.

 If you answered fewer than four questions correctly, that's okay! We'll count this one as warm-up therapy.

5 Therapeutic modalities

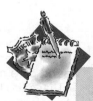

Just the facts

In this chapter, you'll learn:

♦ therapeutic modalities for wound healing

♦ physiological effects of therapeutic modalities

♦ indications, contraindications and application methods for therapeutic modalities.

A look at therapeutic modalities

A wide variety of skin and wound care treatments are available to complement the function of wound dressings. These are commonly described as adjunctive or therapeutic modalities – treatments that are used in addition to standard therapies. (See *How therapeutic modalities promote healing*, page 96.)

Tradition!

Some therapeutic modalities, such as hydrotherapy and therapeutic light, have been used since the early 1900s. Many traditional modalities are still widely used today and new therapeutic modalities are always being developed. Therapeutic modalities, like dressings, should be chosen for their suitability for the patient and the suggested mode of action should be carefully considered before treatment proceeds. It should be noted that use of modalities varies between countries and not all are used in the UK. It is also important to note that for many of the modalities, even those used for many years, there is limited research evidence to support their use in wound care.

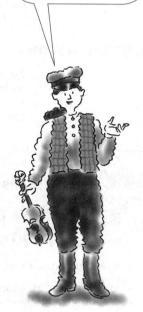

Some therapeutic modalities, such as larval therapy, have been in use for hundreds of years. New treatments, often based on the traditional, continue to emerge.

Common therapeutic modalities

Therapeutic modalities include:
- biotherapy (growth factors, living skin equivalents)
- electrical stimulation
- hydrotherapy
- hyperbaric oxygen
- larval therapy
- non-contact normothermic wound therapy
- pulsed radio signals
- therapeutic light (UV treatment, laser therapy)
- topical negative therapy
- ultrasound.

Selecting a therapeutic modality

To select the best therapeutic modalities for the patient, focus on his specific wound care needs. For example, if the wound needs debridement to remove necrosis and reduce microorganism counts, consider using:
Larval therapy.

Lighten the load

For oedema and lymphoedema control and to reduce pathologic intercellular fluid loads, consider:
- compression bandages or stockings. (See Chapter 10, *Leg ulcers*.)

> Think about your patient's wound care needs. That's the key to selecting the best therapeutic modality for each patient.

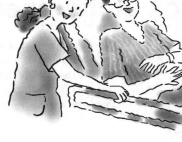

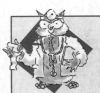

Get wise to wounds

How therapeutic modalities promote healing

Therapeutic modalities promote wound healing by:

- physically or mechanically debriding particulate and bacterial necrosis
- killing or controlling microorganism numbers
- reducing or controlling oedema and wound fluids
- increasing blood flow and tissue oxygenation
- enhancing immune or connective tissue cell function
- providing scaffolding for tissue growth.

Very stimulating!

To stimulate tissue formation by increasing blood vessel formation (angiogenesis); to enhance blood flow and the delivery of oxygen, nutrients and immune cells; to improve immune cell and wound bed cell function; and to stimulate wound matrix formation and collagen fibre alignment, the following might be considered:

- growth factors
- living skin equivalents
- hyperbaric oxygen
- topical negative therapy.

Biotherapy

The biotherapy methods most commonly used in wound treatment include growth factors and living skin equivalents.

Growth factors

Growth factors are an important form of biotherapy because of the important role they play in the healing process (stimulating cell proliferation).

Getting the factors straight

Wound healing is a complex process that the body undertakes to replace or repair injured tissue. If various growth factors aren't synthesised, secreted and removed from tissues with correct timing, the wound healing process can stall. This leaves the wound bed in a chronic state of confusion, unable to heal.

The master factor

In the past decade, growth factors have been studied to determine exactly how they function in healing and how they may be used in the treatment of chronic wounds. (See *Understanding growth factors*, page 98.) Particular focus has been placed on platelet-derived growth factor (PDGF), which some experts call the master factor. Although the specific growth factor or other mechanism that initiates wound healing isn't known, PDGF is known to play a central role by attracting fibroblasts (component of granulation tissue) and inducing them to divide. This is central to wound healing because fibroblasts are responsible for collagen formation.

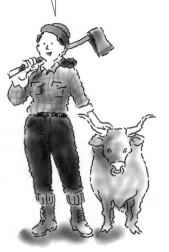

Growth factors stimulate cell proliferation, making them an important component of the healing process.

Understanding growth factors

This chart describes key growth factors that play an important role in wound healing.

Type	Brief description
TGF-β (transforming growth factor beta)	Controls movement of cells to sites of inflammation and stimulates extracellular matrix formation
bFGF (basic fibroblast growth factor)	Stimulates angiogenesis (the development of blood vessels)
VEGF (vascular endothelial growth factor)	Stimulates angiogenesis
IGF (insulin-like growth factor)	Increases collagen synthesis
EGF (epidermal growth factor)	Stimulates epidermal regeneration

Trials and tribulations

The key growth factors PDGF, TGF-β, bFGF and EGF have been through or are currently undergoing testing in clinical trials. An example of a synthetic growth factor approved for use in the UK is becaplermin (Regranex® Gel 0.01%), which has a biological activity similar to that of endogenous PDGF.

Dime-size dynamo

Regranex® is recommended for use on lower-extremity diabetic neuropathic ulcers that have adequate blood flow and involve tissues at and below the subcutaneous level. A small amount is applied to the ulcer using a sterile applicator, the ulcer can then be covered with a sterile secondary dressing such as a foam dressing. Regranex® is contraindicated in necrotic and infected wounds and in patients with poor blood supply to the legs.

A word of caution

An increased risk of mortality secondary to malignancy has been reported in patients using 3 or more tubes of Regranex® (Hart and Rosenthal 2008) and it should therefore be used with caution particularly on patients with known malignancy.

Biological dressings (or living skin equivalents)

Another type of biotherapy available for chronic wound management involves the use of living skin equivalents, also called tissue-engineered skin substitutes.

It's alive!

Living skin equivalents are living constructs derived from biological substances, such as bovine collagen and human neonatal foreskin. All living skin equivalents should be used on wounds with adequate blood flow that are free from infection and necrosis. Living skin equivalent is applied to a clean wound bed and several applications may be needed. This sterile procedure usually requires special training. Be aware that these products are expensive, require special storage, and some have a short half-life. Examples of living skin equivalents include Apligraf® and Dermagraft®, both used in the US.

Living skin equivalents are often made from bovine collagen.

Electrical therapies

Electrical stimulation is used to enhance healing of recalcitrant wounds, especially chronic pressure ulcers. The types of electrical stimulation used in wound healing include high-voltage and low-voltage pulsed current. Electrical stimulation is delivered through a device that has conductive electrodes, which are applied to the skin.

Zap it!

Electrical stimulation can be used to promote healing by:
* promote cellular migration
* enhance blood flow
* increase protein synthesis and wound bed formation
* destroy microorganisms
* increase angiogenesis
* increase tissue oxygenation
* reduce wound bioburden or microbial content
* reduce pain (wound and diabetic neuropathic pain).

Lack of stimulation

Contraindications for electrical stimulation include:
* malignant tissue
* untreated osteomyelitis
* treatment over pericardial area(s) related to control of cardiac and respiratory function
* treatment over implanted electronic devices.

There is research evidence to support the use of electrical therapies in wound care (Kloth 2005) although which approach is best to use is uncertain. An example of an electrical therapy product is POSiFECT® which delivers a battery-powered current to the wound area. This therapy is integrated into a dressing so that the wound is appropriately covered during the treatment period.

Hydrotherapy

Hydrotherapy is used in wound care by a number of different disciplines (such as physical therapy). It is rarely used in the UK and is included here for reference only. Examples of hydrotherapy are:
- pulsatile lavage with concurrent suction
- whirlpool therapy
- jet irrigation.
    As with most treatments, the type of therapy used depends on the patient's wound type.

Pulsatile lavage

Pulsatile lavage cleans and debrides wounds by combining pulse irrigation with suction. It can be used on a number of wound types: acute or chronic, large or small, infected or non-infected and sloughy or necrotic. Suggested advantages of using pulsatile lavage include:
- pressure of lavage can be varied by user
- mobility of the apparatus (can be performed in a hospital, clinic or home setting)
- effectiveness in reaching deep, tunnelling wounds
- minimised chance of cross-contamination.
    However, the procedure can be uncomfortable and therefore patients should be premedicated with an analgesic before starting.
    Pulsatile lavage is rarely used in the UK.

Whirlpool therapy

In whirlpool therapy, part of the patient's body is immersed in a tank of water that has been heated to a prescribed temperature and circulated by an agitator. This therapy softens necrotic tissue, removes debris and exudate and improves blood flow to the area, enhancing the delivery of oxygen and nutrients. Treatment times range from 10 to 20 minutes. A whirlpool tank may also be used for exercise therapy for patients with open wounds or when a therapeutic pool isn't available.
    Indications for whirlpool treatment include:
- large surface area wounds
- wounds with tough, black eschar
- wounds with particulate (such as 'road rash')
- painful wounds.

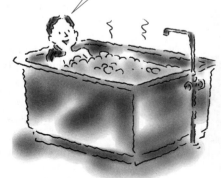

Whirlpool tanks come in several sizes, depending on the area of the body that needs treatment.

Everyone else, out of the pool!

Contraindications to whirlpool include:
- wound infections
- oedema
- deep vein thrombosis or acute phlebitis
- cardiovascular, pulmonary or renal failure

- unresponsiveness or dementia
- bowel or bladder incontinence
- wounds with dry gangrene.

Whirlpool therapy is not widely used in the UK.

Hyperbaric oxygen

Hyperbaric oxygen therapy (HBOT) is the delivery of 100% oxygen through a sealed chamber. Two forms of HBOT are used for wound healing. One form involves a total body chamber, such as that used for decompression therapy for divers, and the other involves a smaller chamber used just for the limbs.

In demand

HBOT delivered by a whole body chamber increases the amount of dissolved oxygen in the blood that's available for wound healing. This increased availability of readily available oxygen in the blood can be used by cells, such as neutrophils, that employ oxygen-dependent processes. (The processes by which neutrophils destroy microorganisms are oxygen-based, as is cellular metabolism in general). In addition, the increased availability of oxygen for tissues apparently relieves relative hypoxia in wounded tissues.

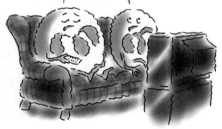

This film is making me feel sleepy, what can I do?

What you need is some hyperbaric oxygen therapy to get you moving again!

Give it a go!

Evidence supporting systemic or whole body HBOT treatment for patients with chronic wounds is evolving. A review of the research indicated benefits for diabetic patients with foot ulcers (Kranke *et al.* 2004). HBOT increases nitric oxide production in the wound. Nitric oxide is a unique free radical that's important in vasodilation and neurotransmission, which play major roles in diabetic wound healing. However, keep in mind that HBOT is contraindicated for patients taking antineoplastic agents or who are experiencing pneumothorax.

HBOT is a modality that is only offered in a few specialist centres around the UK. Patients who may benefit from HBOT are referred to their nearest centre for consideration of suitability.

Larval therapy

Larvae have been used in wound care for many hundreds of years but fell out of use in the early years of the 20th century following the introduction of modern surgical techniques and antibiotics. In recent years their popularity has risen again and the evidence base is growing as to their benefits.

Larval therapy is used for the removal of soft necrotic or sloughy tissue. This involves the use of sterile maggots (from the *Lucilia sericata* fly) which are applied to the wound either in a mesh bag or under a mesh dressing. The larvae are supplied with specialist dressings and advice on the application procedure. When in the wound bed the larvae produce a proteolytic enzyme which liquefies non-viable tissue, this is then ingested as a source of nutrition. The larvae also reduce malodour by ingesting bacteria in the wound bed (Acton 2007).

We're gonna clean this wound up once and for all!

When it is used

Larval therapy can be used in many wound types including pressure ulcers, diabetic ulcers, surgical wounds and burns. Larvae are most effective on soft necrotic tissue (they do not like hard eschar!) and slough. Hard eschar must be softened first with a hydrogel. Be careful to remove the hydrogel thoroughly before applying the larvae as they are killed by the preservatives in many hydrogel-dressing products.

What's the advantage?

Larval therapy is a cost-effective debridement option for patients who are not fit to undergo surgery; 2–3 treatments is usually sufficient to debride the wound bed fully. In addition

- larvae do not harm healthy tissue
- they usually debride more quickly than conventional dressings
- they are thought to stimulate granulation tissue (Prete 1997).

Considerations

You must clearly explain what larvae therapy involves (the use of live maggots) and ensure your patient fully understands what will happen. It is good practice to obtain written consent prior to commencing treatment. In addition, you should explain that:

- the movement of the larvae in the wound bed can sometimes be felt
- the initial activity of the larvae results in an increase in wound exudate during the first 24–48 hours and that this is a normal consequence of the debridement activity
- any pain or bleeding should be reported to the nurse or clinician in charge.

Leave them out

Larvae should not be applied to wounds that have a tendency to bleed or to any large blood vessels. They should not be introduced into wounds that communicate with a body cavity or internal organ.

Non-contact normothermic wound therapy

Non-contact normothermic wound therapy (NNWT) is a temporary therapy that increases the temperature of the wound bed. This is intended to promote increased blood flow in the area of the wound. An example of this therapy is the Warm-Up™ Therapy System, which comprises a dressing with an integral electronic warming card. Once in place, the card heats to 38° C, bathing the wound in radiant heat. The closely sealed wound covering promotes a moist environment in the wound bed. This system is designed to remain in place for 72 hours.

When it's used

It can be used on acute or chronic, full-thickness or partial-thickness wounds, regardless of aetiology, that have failed to heal with traditional therapies, including wounds with compromised blood flow, such as arterial or diabetic foot ulcers.

What's the advantage?

The Warm-Up™ Therapy System can absorb a small-to-moderate amount of drainage in the wound covering. In addition, it doesn't disturb the wound when removed and can be used on infected wounds.

What to consider

The Warm-Up™ Therapy System is contraindicated for use on third-degree burns. In addition, it requires specific dressings and thorough patient teaching related to dressing changes and heat management.

Research evidence supporting the use of this therapy is limited at present.

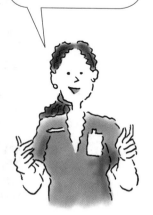

The Warm-Up Therapy System increases the temperature of the wound bed, which increases blood flow in the wound area.

Pulsed radio signals

The Provant® Wound Therapy System is a non-invasive treatment that is reported to aid in the reduction of pain and swelling of the skin and soft tissues following surgery. It does this by sending a pulsed radio signal into the tissues around the wound.

Clinical studies indicate that the Provant® system might promote healing, even in cases of chronic, severe pressure ulcers (Ritz *et al.* 2002). The radio frequency stimuli Provant® uses is thought to induce the proliferation of fibroblasts and epithelial cells in the injured area.

When it's used

Use the Provant® Wound Therapy System on wounds in the inflammatory phase of healing.

What's the advantage?

The Provant® Wound Therapy System:
•   requires minimal training (patients may be able to perform therapy at home)
•   requires two 30-minute treatments per day (duration is pre-set in the device so it turns off automatically at the end of a session)
•   may be used over existing dressings.

What to consider

The Provant® system:
- is not indicated for treatment of deep tissue and bone
- should not be used on patients with metallic implants in the area of application
- should not be used on patients with cardiac pacemakers
- should not be used during patient pregnancy
- should not be used over the joints of patients with immature bone development.

Research supporting the use of this therapy is limited at present and it is rarely used in the UK.

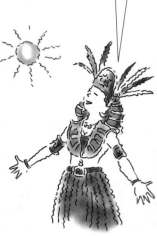

Light therapy is as old as the sun.

Therapeutic light

In therapeutic light modalities, light or its energy is used to aid in wound healing. The modalities include UV treatment and laser therapy.

UV treatment

Although not a form of light, UV energy or radiation is commonly categorised as therapeutic light. UV energy lies between X-rays and visible light on the electromagnetic spectrum. It has been used for more than 100 years for the treatment of slow healing and infected wounds. Heliotherapy, or sun therapy, has been used for thousands of years for skin problems and other healthcare needs.

Strike up the bands

UV radiation is typically divided into three bands: UVA, UVB and UVC. Here are some of the suggested benefits of treatment with UVA and UVB radiation:
- UVA and UVB energy enhances WBC accumulation and lysosomal activity, possibly offering an explanation for UV-mediated debridement.
- UV radiation stimulates the production of interleukin-1 alpha, a cytokine that plays a role in epithelialisation.

UV utility

Indications for UV treatment include:
- chronic, slow healing wounds
- infected or heavily contaminated wounds
- necrotic wounds.

Contraindications for UV treatment include certain chronic disease states, such as:
- diabetes
- pulmonary tuberculosis
- hyperthyroidism

- systemic lupus erythematosus
- cardiac disease
- renal disease
- hepatic disease
- acute eczema
- herpes simplex.
  In the UK, UV treatment is used in skin care but rarely on wounds.

Laser therapy

The word 'laser' is actually an acronym for light amplification by stimulated emission of radiation. Lasers can be divided into two groups:
- Cold lasers include the helium neon, or red laser, and the gallium arsenide laser.
- Hot lasers encompass the carbon dioxide laser and other lasers used for surgical dissection.

In wound healing, cold low-level lasers are used to promote wound closure and nerve regeneration. The treatment consists of either placing the laser probe directly over selected treatment points for a specific time, according to the dosage required, or using a grid-like pattern and continuously moving the probe over this grid for a specific treatment time.

Laser tag

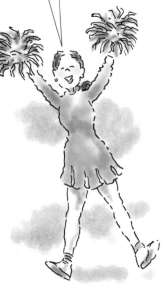

Gimme an L!
Gimme an A!
Gimme an S-E-R!
What does it spell?
LASER! What does it stand for?
Light amplification by stimulated emission of radiation!

Indications for cold low-level laser therapy include:
- slow healing wounds
- nerve regeneration
- pain relief.
  Contraindications for cold low-level laser therapy include treatments over:
- the eye
- a haemorrhage
- a malignancy
- a pregnant woman's uterus
- photosensitive skin.

A systematic review of the literature concluded that there was no evidence of any benefit associated with low-level laser therapy on venous leg ulcer healing (Flemming and Cullum 1999). There remains limited evidence to support the use of this modality in these or any other types of wound.

Topical negative pressure therapy

Topical negative pressure (TNP) therapy uses negative air pressure to promote wound closure. It can be used when a wound fails to heal in a timely manner. A number of manufacturers make TNP devices. The KCI system, called VAC®, consists of a special open-cell polyurethane ether foam dressing cut to the size of the wound, a vacuum tube and a vacuum pump. One end of the vacuum tube is placed over the foam dressing and the other connects to the vacuum pump. The dressing is sealed securely in place with an adhesive film dressing that extends 3 to 5 cm over adjacent skin all around the foam. The Talley system, called Venturi®, consists of a silicone drain, specially designed gauze and an adhesive film dressing. The gauze (sometimes moistened with saline) is placed in the wound cavity and the silicone drain positioned on it, the whole wound is then covered with the transparent dressing. The drain is attached to the vacuum pump. Both systems have disposable drainage cannisters attached to the pumps.

When turned on, the vacuum pumps gently reduce air pressure beneath the dressing, drawing off exudate and reducing oedema in surrounding tissues. This process reduces bacterial colonisation, promotes granulation tissue development, increases the rate of cell mitosis and spurs the migration of epithelial cells within the wound. Many clinicians report favourable results when using TNP, however, a Cochrane Review advised that research into its benefits is inconclusive and that better quality evidence was needed to support this modality (Ubbink *et al.* 2007).

Mini-me

Portable devices are also available. These smaller models run on rechargeable batteries and their drainage capacity is much smaller.

When it's used

TNP therapy is useful in managing slow-healing acute, sub-acute, or chronic exudative wounds with cavities. It can be used on cavity wounds such as pressure ulcers or surgical wounds and on relatively flat wounds such as venous leg ulcers.

What's the advantage?

TNP:
- cleans deeply and can manage moderate-to-large amounts of drainage
- can manage multiple wounds when dressings are cut to bridge two or more wounds (or when a Y-connector connects two wounds to one unit)
- the portable units have rechargeable batteries and are small enough to fit in a pouch that can be worn at the waist or over the shoulder (e.g. VAC Freedom®).

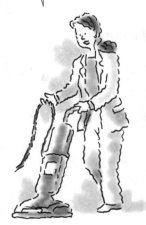

It's time to get the vacuum going on this wound.

Topical negative therapy

TNP therapy encourages healing by applying localised sub-atmospheric pressure at the site of the wound. This reduces oedema and bacterial colonisation and stimulates the formation of granulation tissue. This illustration shows the components of a VAC therapy device.

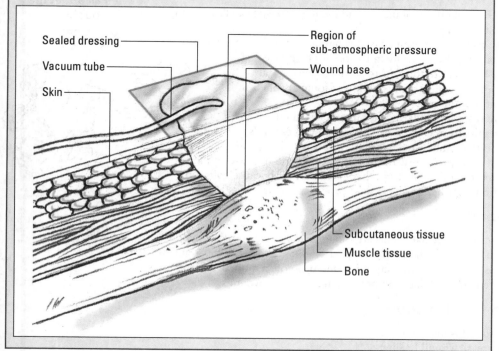

Sealed dressing

Vacuum tube

Skin

Region of sub-atmospheric pressure

Wound base

Subcutaneous tissue

Muscle tissue

Bone

What to consider

Training is required to ensure TNP is used correctly and with maximum effect.

TNP therapy is contraindicated for use with untreated osteomyelitis, malignancies and wounds with necrotic tissue or fistulas. In addition:
• the TNP tubing requires that the patient remain in one place or carry the unit along, the pump units are quite heavy
• permanent devices require electricity; the portable versions must be recharged frequently
• incorrect use of TNP, such as improperly setting the pump pressure, can result in bruising at the wound base and pain.

TNP is popular in the UK with many organisations owning or leasing systems on a regular basis.

Ultrasound

Ultrasound (mechanical pressure waves) is used in treatments for patients with both open and closed wounds because of its non-thermal and thermal effects.

Cavitation sensation

Non-thermal effects of ultrasound include acoustic cavitation and microstreaming.
• In acoustic cavitation, gaseous bubbles are made to expand and contract rhythmically in the tissues being treated. These bubbles are thought to stimulate biological phenomena such as the activation of ionic channels in cellular membranes.
• Microstreaming is another non-thermal effect that results from cavitation. Cavitation causes fluids close to the bubbles to stream by, thus stimulating the cells in close proximity. In this way, ultrasound increases calcium conductance in fibroblasts, which is important because collagen secretion is a calcium-dependent process.

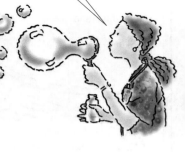

Ultrasound aids wound healing non-thermally through acoustic cavitation and microstreaming. It's all about the bubbles.

Gets the blood flowing

Ultrasound's thermal effects are thought to include increased blood flow to tissue, which results in increased tissue healing. Ultrasound may also increase WBC migration and promote a more orderly arrangement of collagen in both open and closed wounds.

This might be a job for ultrasound

Ultrasound is indicated to:
• increase wound healing
• enhance blood flow
• decrease pain
• decrease inflammation.
  Contraindications for ultrasound include:
• malignant tissue
• acute infections
• deep vein thrombosis
• ischaemic areas
• plastic implants or implanted electronic devices
• irradiated areas
• treatment over the gonads, spinal cord, eyes or a pregnant woman's uterus.
    A systematic review of the research in support of ultrasound in the treatment of pressure ulcers found little evidence of benefit (Baba-Akbari Sari et al. 2006) although the lack of evidence both for or against was acknowledged.

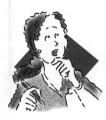

Quick quiz

1. Which growth factor is marketed as Regranex®?
   A. TGF-β
   B. PDGF
   C. IGF
   D. VEGF.

Answer: B. Becaplermin (Regranex® Gel 0.01%) which has a biological activity similar to that of PDGF produced by the body.

2. Which type of therapy increases the amount of dissolved oxygen in the blood?
   A. ultrasound
   B. electrical stimulation
   C. laser
   D. HBOT.

Answer: D. By increasing the amount of dissolved oxygen in the blood, HBOT therapy increases the availability of oxygen to wounded tissues, which improves healing.

3. Which condition is contraindicated for the use of electrical stimulation?
   A. untreated osteomyelitis
   B. chronic pressure ulcers
   C. decreased tissue oxygenation
   D. decreased blood flow.

Answer: A. Electrical stimulation is contraindicated for a patient with untreated osteomyelitis.

4. What is the Latin name of the fly used in larvae therapy?
   A. *Calliphora vomitoria*
   B. *Chrysops relictus*
   C. *Lucilia sericata*
   D. *Tsetse.*

Answer: C. *Lucilia sericata*, commonly known as the greenbottle fly.

5. What kind of waves are ultrasound?
   A. pressure waves
   B. radio waves
   C. pushing waves
   D. pulsating waves.

Answer: A. Pressure waves.

6. Which wound care product uses negative pressure to promote wound closure?
   A.　TNP therapy
   B.　Warm-Up Therapy System
   C.　debriding agent
   D.　hydrocolloid dressing.

Answer:　A. TNP (topical negative pressure therapy) devices generate negative pressure that draw off exudate and promote granulation.

Scoring

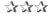 If you answered all six questions correctly, take a bow! You're sizzling hot when it comes to therapeutic modalities.

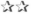 If you answered four to five questions correctly, don't give up! Time and a quick review will heal your wounded pride.

 If you answered fewer than four questions correctly, maybe you whirled through the information too quickly! Review the chapter and try again.

References

Acton, C. (2007) A know-how guide to using larval therapy for wound debridement. *Wound Essentials* 2:156–159.

Baba-Akbari Sari, A., Flemming, K., Cullum, N.A. *et al.* (2006) Therapeutic ultrasound for pressure ulcers. *Cochrane Database of Systematic Reviews.* Issue 3.

Flemming, K. and Cullum, N. (1999) Laser therapy for venous leg ulcers. *Cochrane Database of Systematic Reviews.* Issue 1.

Hart, J.C. and Rosenthal, N. (2008) Important drug warning – Regranex®. Ortho-McNeil Janssen Pharmaceuticals. [on-line] [Accessed 23 August 2008] Available: http://www.regranex.com/

Kloth, L.C. (2005) Electrical stimulation for wound healing: a review of evidence from in-vitro studies, animal experiments and clinical trials. *International Journal of Lower Extremities* 4(1):23–44.

Kranke, P., Bennett, M., Roeckl-Wiedmann, I. *et al.* (2004) Hyperbaric oxygen therapy for chronic wounds. *Cochrane Database of Systematic Reviews.* Issue 2

Prete, P. (1997) Growth effects of Phaenicia sericata larval extracts on fibroblasts: mechanism for wound healing by maggot therapy. *Life Sciences* 60(8):505–510.

Ritz, M.C., Gallegos, R., Canham, M.B. *et al.* (2002) Provant® wound-closure system accelerates closure of pressure wounds in a randomised, double blind, placebo-controlled trial. *Annals of the New York Academy of Science* 961:356–359.

Ubbink, D.T., Westerbos, S.J., Evans, D. *et al.* (2007) Topical negative pressure for treating chronic wounds. *Cochrane Database of Systematic Reviews.* Issue 4.

6 Acute wounds

Just the facts

In this chapter, you'll learn:

♦ types of acute wounds, including those caused by surgery, trauma and burns

♦ assessment factors for each type of acute wound

♦ ways in which skin grafts are used to repair defects caused by acute wounds.

A look at acute wounds

Three criteria are generally used to classify wounds and determine their severity: age, depth and colour. However, to determine a wound's age, you must first determine if it's acute or chronic. To do this, you shouldn't adhere solely to a timeline; you should also consider the wound's progress towards healing. Ask these questions when characterising an acute wound:

• Is the wound new or relatively new?
• Did the wound occur suddenly (as opposed to developing over time)?
• Is the wound healing in a timely, predictable and measurable manner?

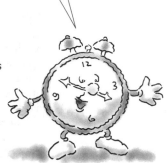

Time isn't the only distinguishing factor when determining whether a wound is acute or chronic.

Intent or accident?

Acute wounds can occur by intention or trauma. For example, a surgical incision is an acute wound that's caused intentionally. Traumatic (accidental) wounds have a wide variety of causes including abrasions, lacerations, skin tears and bites. Traumatic wounds inflicted by self harming are caused with intention and range from simple to severe. Burns are a category of traumatic wound that have a unique set of causes, potential complications and treatment options.

Regardless of the cause, when caring for a patient with an acute wound, you'll focus on restoring normal anatomical structure, physiological function and appearance to the wound area (sometimes accomplished by skin grafting). You will also need to be aware of any psychosocial factors influencing the progress of the wound and the patient's general well-being. (See Chapter 7, *Psychosocial effects*, page 151.)

Surgical wounds

An acute surgical wound is a healthy and uncomplicated break in the skin's continuity resulting from surgery. In an otherwise healthy individual, this type of wound responds well to postoperative care and heals without incident in a predictable period of time.

Factors that affect healing

Several factors can greatly affect the course of postoperative wound healing. These include the patient's age, nutritional status, general health before surgery and oxygenation status.

Age

Age is an important factor in the healing process, especially for paediatric patients and older adults. Premature infants and infants up to age 1 have immature immune systems and are therefore at greater risk for infection before, during and after surgery. At the other end of the age continuum, older adults commonly have a harder time healing after surgery due to skin changes. (See *Age and wound healing*, page 113.)

Nutrition

Proper nutrition is crucial for the body to heal itself effectively. During the preoperative assessment, it's imperative to identify nutritional problems early and to develop a plan that addresses deficits.

After surgery, the body quickly depletes its stores of nutrients (especially in the highly exudative wound) and even an otherwise healthy patient can become malnourished if diet is ignored. The care plan must include a diet with adequate nutrients and fluids to create an optimum environment for wound healing.

Because the body quickly depletes its nutrient stores after surgery, be sure to include a balanced diet with adequate nutrients in your care plan.

Handle with care

Age and wound healing

In infants and elderly patients, surgical wounds may not heal normally.

Infants

In premature infants and infants up to age 1, the immune system and other body systems aren't fully developed, so there's a greater risk for infection before, during and after surgery. Sterile (aseptic) technique is a critical component of care for very young patients.

Elderly patients

Skin becomes thinner and less elastic with age. Populations of cells that repair tissues and fight infection decline and the skin's vascular system is less robust. As a result, surgical wounds in elderly patients heal more slowly, increasing the risk of infection.

Adipose poses problems

A patient who's overweight has an additional problem. Adipose tissue lacks the extensive vascular supply present in skin. As the amount of adipose tissue increases, blood flow to the skin decreases. This reduces the amount of oxygen and nutrients reaching the wound area, which impedes healing and increases the risk of wound dehiscence.

Illness

In most cases, a pre-existing illness or infection delays or complicates healing after surgery. Unfortunately, it isn't always possible to delay surgery while an underlying condition resolves itself. In these cases, the care plan must include measures that minimise the impact of the pre-existing condition on the healing process. For example:
•   Disorders that impede blood flow, such as coronary artery disease, peripheral vascular disease (PVD) and hypertension, can cause problems by reducing the flow of blood reaching the incision site. A patient with one of these conditions requires a care plan that includes interventions to improve circulation.
•   Cancer may necessitate more aggressive pain management or a care plan that includes management of symptoms such as nausea and vomiting.

• Diabetes mellitus impedes healing in many ways and increases the patient's risk of infection. Diabetic neuropathy (inflammation and degeneration of peripheral nerves), if present, can interfere with vasodilation and, consequently, circulation in the area of the incision.

• Immunosuppression resulting from either a disease or drug therapy (corticosteroids, chemotherapy) may impair the inflammatory response, delaying wound healing and increasing the patient's risk of infection.

Surgical site infection

Wound infections that occur at the site of a surgical incision, i.e. postoperatively, are referred to as surgical site infections (SSIs). SSIs are one of the most important causes of healthcare-associated infections (HCAIs) in the UK (NICE 2008). In one study, nearly 5% of surgical patients were found to have an SSI (Smyth 2006). The most common time for an SSI to develop is between the 5th and 10th day post-operatively (NICE 2008). Prompt recognition of SSI is vital to minimise the risk of further complications developing such as wound dehiscence and septicaemia.

Three levels of SSI have been described (NICE 2008, Horan *et al.* 1992):

• Superficial incisional, affecting the skin and subcutaneous tissue. Signs include redness, pain, heat or swelling at the site of the incision, drainage of pus.

• Deep incisional, affecting the fascial and muscle layers. Signs include pus or abscess, fever with tenderness of the wound, separation of the edges of the incision exposing the deeper tissues.

• Organ or space infection, involving any part of the anatomy other than the incision, that is opened or manipulated during the surgical procedure e.g. joint or peritoneum. Signs include drainage of pus or the formation of an abscess.

(See also Chapter 2, *Recognising infection*, page 40.)

Check your patient regularly for these signs and ask them to report any increasing tenderness or pain in the wound area. Do not disturb the wound dressing unless necessary e.g. wound drainage leaks through the dressing, bleeding is evident, your patient reports increasing tenderness or pain. If clinical signs of infection are present send a wound swab for investigation (see Chapter 3, *Wound specimen collection*, page 77) and report concerns to the surgical team, tissue viability and infection control nurse specialists.

Did you hear that? Some drugs cause immunosuppression, which delays wound healing and increases the risk of infection.

Oxygenation status

Adequate oxygenation is critical to the healing process. During healing, neutrophils require oxygen to produce the hydrogen peroxide they use to kill pathogens, and fibroblasts require oxygen for collagen proliferation. Any condition that impedes overall oxygenation or the amount of oxygen reaching the wound – smoking, for example – slows the healing process. Smoking has a number of consequences including a decreased proportion of circulating oxyhaemoglobin, reduced tissue blood flow and reduced immune response (Ahn *et al*. 2008).

Smoking a single cigarette can lead to transient decrease in skin blood flow regardless of smoking habit, and habitual smokers show delayed recovery of blood flow.

Patient understanding

Your patient should be made aware of how they can help themselves. Preoperative advice on matters such as nutrition and smoking may reduce the risks of postoperative complications; this advice is often given at a pre-surgery assessment clinic but should also be reinforced on admission. It is also important to educate your patient in infection control matters. Explain that they shouldn't interfere with their surgical wound because they will increase the risk of wound infection and explain why hand-washing is important for them and for all the healthcare team caring for them.

Assessment and care

Your care should focus on keeping the wound clean and protecting it from trauma. The exact care required during healing depends on the wound closure method, the development of the healing ridge and the type of dressing ordered. The patient's ability to properly perform wound care after discharge also affects healing.

Wound closure

The surgeon determines the appropriate method of wound closure based on the wound's severity; in most cases, sutures or clips (skin staples) are used.

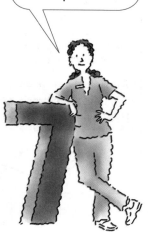

Sutures typically remain in place for 7 to 10 days, as long as no complications are present.

Sew . . . a needle pulling thread

In suturing, a natural or synthetic thread is used to stitch the wound closed. (See *Suture materials and methods*, page 116.)

Sutures typically remain in place for 7 to 10 days, depending on the wound's severity, the type of tissue involved and whether healing is progressing as expected. Factors that affect the timing of suture

Suture materials and methods

When closing a surgical wound, the choice of suture material varies according to the suturing method, location and tissue type.

Materials

Non-absorbable sutures:

- are used to close the skin surface
- provide strength and immobility
- cause minimal tissue irritation
- are made of silk, cotton, stainless steel or Dacron.

  Absorbable sutures:

- are used when suture removal is undesirable (for example, sutures in an underlying tissue layer)
- are made of chromic catgut (a natural catgut treated with chromium trioxide to improve strength and prolong absorption time), plain catgut (a material that's absorbed faster and is more likely to cause irritation than chromic catgut) or synthetic materials (such as polyglycolic acid) that are replacing catgut because they're stronger, more durable and less irritating.

Methods

The most common suture methods include mattress continuous suture, plain continuous suture, mattress interrupted suture, plain interrupted suture and blanket continuous suture.

Mattress continuous suture

Connected mattress stitches with a knot at the beginning and end.

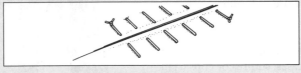

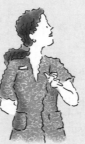

Plain continuous suture

Connected stitches with the thread knotted at the beginning and end of the suture (also called a continuous running suture).

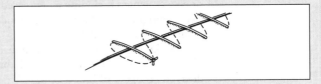

Mattress interrupted suture

Independent stitches with both threads crossing beneath the suture line, leaving only a small portion of suture exposed on each side of the wound.

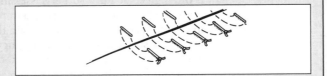

Plain interrupted suture

Individual sutures sewn with a separate piece of thread. Half the thread length crosses under the suture line and the other half crosses above the skin surface.

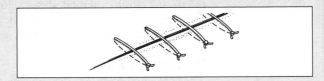

Blanket continuous suture

Looped stitches with a knot at the beginning and end.

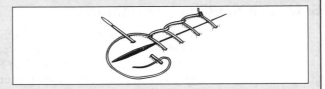

removal include the patient's overall condition; the shape, size and location of the incision; and whether inflammation, drainage or infection develops.

Stainless steel solutions

The surgeon may choose to use clips (skin staples) as an alternative to sutures if cosmetic results aren't an issue. These closures secure a wound faster than sutures and, because they're made of surgical stainless steel, tissue reaction is minimal. Properly placed staples and clips distribute tension evenly along the suture line, reducing tissue trauma and compression. This promotes healing and minimises scarring. The surgeon won't usually use clips if less than 5 mm of tissue exists between the staple and any underlying bone, vessel or organ. (See *Using retention sutures*.)

Stick with me!

Smaller wounds with little drainage can be closed with adhesive skin closures, such as Steri-Strips™ or butterfly closures. As with staples and clips, these closures cause little tissue reaction. Adhesive closures can also be used after suture or staple removal to provide ongoing support for a healing incision. (See *Types of adhesive skin closures*, page 118.) Tissue adhesives (glue) may also be used. (See *Closing up*, page 126.)

The healing ridge

To properly assess healing, it's important to understand how the healing ridge develops in an incision after surgery. The healing ridge is a build-up of collagen fibres that begins to form during the inflammatory phase of wound healing, usually the first 24 to 72 hours. It peaks during the proliferation phase, usually between days 5 and 9 (Bryant and Nix 2006). You should feel this ridge as you gently palpate the skin on each side of the wound. The healing

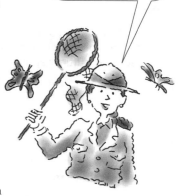

Butterfly closures can be used to promote healing after suture removal.

Handle with care

Using retention sutures

Retention sutures can be used to secure wound edges and to support the suture line. The use of retention sutures for obese patients helps support the deep tissues while the more superficial fascia and skin tissues heal. Retention sutures are placed through the abdominal wall before the abdominal layers are closed to reinforce the suture line.

Types of adhesive skin closures

The two most common types of adhesive skin closures are Steri-Strips and butterfly closures.

Steri-Strips

Steri-Strips™ (thin strips of sterile, non-woven tape) are a primary means of holding a wound closed after suture removal.

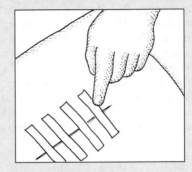

Butterfly closures

Butterfly closures have two sterile, waterproof adhesive strips linked by a narrow, non-adhesive 'bridge'. They're used to hold small wounds closed to promote healing after suture removal.

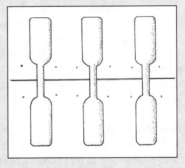

ridge is a sign that healing is progressing. If you can't feel the ridge, healing isn't progressing as expected and further assessment is required. You should notify the surgical team as there is a risk of wound dehiscence.

Dressings

The incision dressing shields the wound against pathogens and protects the skin surface from irritating drainage. The dressing is the primary aspect of wound management for surgical wounds; therefore, choosing the right type is important.

Proper dress required

Typically, lightly exuding closed wounds require an adhesive, low absorbency island dressing; this will suffice until wound drainage ceases 1–2 days postoperatively. Wounds with copious, excoriating exudate require a more absorbent dressing, such as an alginate or a hydrofibre. Alternatively, a wound drainage bag or pouch can be used to collect the exudate and protect the surrounding skin. (See *Applying a wound drainage bag*.) Wound drainage bags also allow for measurement of exudate loss.

When dressing a surgical wound, use sterile technique and sterile supplies to prevent contamination. Change the dressing as often as needed to absorb drainage and keep the surrounding skin dry; however, remember that a wound heals best at body temperature (Lock 1979). Changing the dressing lowers the temperature at the wound site, which slows healing until the site returns to normal body temperature.

Get wise to wounds

Applying a wound drainage bag

If your patient's wound is draining heavily or if drainage may damage surrounding skin, you need to apply a wound drainage bag (pouch). Here's how:

- Measure the wound. Cut an opening 1 cm larger than the wound in the facing of the collection bag (see photo below).

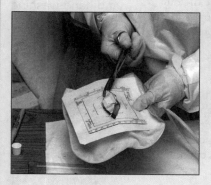

- Apply a skin protectant as needed. (Some protectants are incorporated into the collection bag system and also provide adhesion.)

- Be sure to close the drainage port at the bottom of the bag to prevent leaks. Then gently press the contoured bag opening around the wound, starting at the lower edge, to catch any drainage (see photo below).

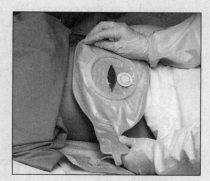

- To empty the bag, put on gloves. Insert the lower portion of the bag into a biohazard container and open the drainage port (see photo top right). Note the colour, consistency, odour and amount of fluid. If ordered, obtain a culture specimen

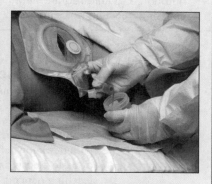

and send it to the laboratory immediately. (Always follow your local infection control policy for handling infectious drainage.)
- Use a gauze pad to wipe the bottom of the bag and the drainage port. This prevents skin irritation or possible odour from any residual drainage. Reseal the port.
- Change the bag only if it leaks or fails to adhere. More frequent changes are unnecessary and can irritate the patient's skin.

Teaching about surgical wound care

Surgical patients need to know the ways that they can promote healing and prevent infection. Be sure to discuss:

- signs and symptoms of wound infection to report to the nurse immediately, such as increased tenderness, deep or increased pain at the wound site, fever or oedema (especially if it occurs between postoperative days 3 and 5)
- how to take an accurate temperature reading
- proper wound care, such as the importance of keeping the incision clean and dry; proper hand-washing technique; and the supplies and methods used to clean the wound
- wound dressings, including the type, where to obtain them and how to open and apply them
- types and levels of permissible activity, such as lifting restrictions (if applicable), when the patient may shower or bathe, and when he can expect to return to work
- nutrition and fluid requirements for healing
- smoking cessation.

Patient education

Patient education is an important component of the care plan for patients with surgical wounds. By the time he's discharged, the patient needs to understand – and demonstrate – the ability to perform proper wound care. Start with an assessment of the patient's knowledge. Then begin your teaching with a discussion of basic asepsis and hand-washing techniques. The balance of your teaching depends on the type of surgery, the type of dressing and the location of the wound. (See *Teaching about surgical wound care.*)

Potential complications

Surgery results in a controlled form of acute wound. The patient's environment, the type and severity of the wound and preoperative and postoperative care are all under the control of the healthcare team. Consequently, most surgical wounds heal without incident; however, some complications that might arise include infection, haemorrhage, dehiscence and evisceration.

Infection

Wound infection is the most common wound complication as well as the third most common hospital acquired infection in the UK (Smyth *et al.* 2008). Preventing wound infection requires meticulous attention to sterile technique when creating and caring for an acute wound.

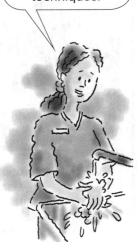

Start patient teaching with the basics – asepsis and hand-washing techniques.

Handle with care

Acute wound complications in patients with morbid obesity (BMI > 40)

Morbidly obese patients are at an increased risk for acute wound complications, including infection, dehiscence caused by increased tension on wound edges at the time of wound closure, and haematoma formation caused by pooled blood.

These complications may be the result of many factors, including:

- difficulty level of operating on these patients
- lengthier operation time, which increases the chances of contamination
- increased trauma (for example, the more forceful retraction needed during surgery may cause necrosis of the abdominal wall).

Mean to intervene

For a surgical patient, wound infection is a significant and serious event requiring prompt intervention. Interventions for post-operative infection include:

- obtaining a wound specimen for culture and sensitivity test
- administering systemic antibiotics
- irrigating the wound with sterile normal saline (0.9%)
- dressing the wound/loosely filling the cavity with an absorbent dressing
- monitoring wound drainage
- providing analgesia.

Haemorrhage

Haemorrhage may occur from damage to blood vessels. In the postoperative patient, it may happen in either internal or external sites. The most common locations of significant internal haemorrhages are:

- posterior nasal passages
- pulmonary vessels
- spleen
- liver
- stomach
- uterus.

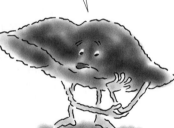

I'm one of the most common locations of post-operative internal haemorrhage. Yikes!

Haemorrhage may also occur at the site of a large artery injury or aneurysm. Haemorrhage in one of these areas significantly reduces the volume of circulating blood and precipitates hypovolaemia. Nursing interventions include administering I.V. fluids to increase blood pressure and urine output and determining the source of bleeding. If the haemorrhage originates externally – for example, from the wound itself or from damage to the fragile, newly developed blood vessels – place pressure or a pressure dressing on the site of the bleeding and notify the surgical team for further advice.

Dehiscence and evisceration

Dehiscence may occur when infection disrupts the healing wound, when there is excessive strain on the incision site or when the new collagen fibres are too weak or immature to hold the wound together. The first sign of dehiscence may be an abscess or a gush of serosanguineous fluid from the wound or a report from the patient of a 'popping' sensation after sneezing, coughing or retching. Complete dehiscence leads to evisceration, in which underlying tissues protrude through the wound opening. Abdominal wounds are more likely to dehisce and eviscerate than thoracic wounds.

An ounce of prevention

Successful wound healing relies on oxygen and nutrients being delivered to the wound bed. The levels delivered are dependent on there being a good blood supply to the wound bed with minimal tissue oedema. Failure in any of these areas will affect the healing process and increase the potential for dehiscence. Malnourishment for example can lead to increased risk of infection and subsequent wound breakdown (Myers 2004) whilst protein deficiency can lead to decreased tensile strength and wound dehiscence (Linblad 1998). In some cases the presence of disease such as diabetes or the long term use of drugs such as corticosteriods, can affect the healing process and again increase the risk of dehiscence (Benbow 2005).

To prevent wound dehiscence and evisceration, ensure your patient receives a well balanced diet preoperatively and postoperatively, discourage them from smoking, observe aseptic procedures where appropriate and teach them to support the incision with a pillow or cushion before they change position, cough or sneeze. Some patients, those who are obese for example, may also require an abdominal support.

If dehiscence occurs, take these steps:
• Stay with the patient; keep him still and have a colleague notify the surgical team on call.

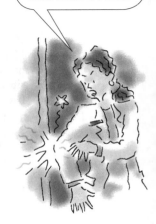

Ouch! It may not seem too traumatic, but even a minor abrasion such as a skinned elbow is considered a traumatic wound.

- If the patient has an abdominal wound, help them into a low Fowler's position, with their knees bent to reduce abdominal tension.
- If evisceration is evident, cover extruding tissues with large sterile dressing pads saturated with sterile normal saline (0.9%).

Traumatic wounds

A traumatic wound is a sudden injury to the skin that can range from minor (such as a skinned knee) to severe (such as a gunshot wound). It includes those wounds caused by non-accidental injury and self harming.

Types of traumatic wounds

Traumatic wounds include abrasions, lacerations, skin tears, bites and penetrating trauma wounds.

Abrasions
An abrasion occurs when a mechanical force, such as friction or shearing, scrapes away a partial thickness of the skin. Unless an unusually large amount of skin is involved or an infection develops, an abrasion is one of the least complicated traumatic wounds.

Lacerations
A laceration is a tear in the skin that's caused by a sharp object, such as metal, glass or wood. It can also be caused by trauma that produces high shearing force. A laceration has jagged, irregular edges and its severity depends on its cause, size, depth and location.

Skin tears
A skin tear is a specific type of laceration that most often affects older adults. In a skin tear, friction alone – or shearing force plus friction – separates layers of skin. A partial-thickness wound occurs if the epidermis separates from the dermis; a full-thickness wound occurs if the epidermis and dermis separate from underlying tissue. Use a classification system, such as Payne–Martin (Payne and Martin 1993), to classify skin tears during assessment. (See *Classifying skin tears*.) This type of injury may be preventable through careful handling by members of the healthcare team. (See *Preventing skin tears*, page 124.)

> ## Classifying skin tears
>
> To provide consistent assessment of skin tears, utilise a classification system such as the Payne–Martin system to document your findings.
>
> The Payne–Martin system classifies skin tears as:
>
> - Category I – skin tear without tissue loss
> - Category II – skin tear with partial tissue loss
> - Category III – skin tear with complete tissue loss, in which the epidermal flap is absent.

Preventing skin tears

As ageing occurs, the skin becomes more prone to skin tear injuries. Prevent skin tears by using:

- proper moving, handling, transferring and repositioning techniques to reduce or eliminate friction or shear
- padding on support surfaces where the risk is greatest, such as bed rails and limb supports on a wheelchair, and over skin when limb restraints are used
- pillows or cushions to support the patient's arms and legs
- non-adherent dressings or those with minimal adherence such as paper tape
- a skin protection wipe before applying dressings
- the push–pull technique to cautiously remove tape or other adhesives in the direction of hair growth
- wraps, such as a stockinette or soft gauze, to protect areas of skin where the risk of tearing is high
- moisturiser to dry skin

Be sure to tell your patient to:

- add protection by wearing long-sleeved shirts and long trousers, weather permitting
- avoid sudden or brusque movements that can pull the skin and possibly cause a skin tear.

Bites

When assessing a bite wound, it's important to quickly discover the bite's source – cat, dog, snake, spider, human? This helps the health-care team determine which bacteria or toxins may be present and the likely type of tissue trauma.

Fancy a bite?

For example, a human bite can cause a puncture wound and introduce any one of the innumerable organisms present in the human mouth into the wound. *Staphylococcus aureus* and *streptococci species* are two such organisms that can be transmitted to the wound or into the victim's bloodstream. Other serious diseases that can be transmitted in this way include HIV infection, hepatitis B, hepatitis C, syphilis and tuberculosis. Some evidence (Wienert *et al.* 1999) suggests that a human bite can also cause necrotising fasciitis (a rapidly progressing and often fatal soft tissue infection).

Animal house

A bite from a dog, cat or rodent can introduce deadly infectious diseases, such as rabies, into a wound. Cats and other smaller mammals cause relatively little tissue damage. However, a dog can generate up to 200 psi of pressure when biting and if they shake their head at the same time (which is usually the case), strong torsional force is brought to bear. Together, these forces can cause a massive amount of tissue damage.

Penetrating trauma wounds

A penetrating trauma wound is a puncture wound. This type of wound may be the result of an accident or a personal attack, as in the case of a stabbing or gunshot wound.

Knife strife

A stab wound is a low-velocity wound that generally presents as a classic puncture wound or laceration. In some cases, it may involve organ damage beneath the wound site. X-rays, computerised tomography scanning and magnetic resonance imaging (MRI) are used to evaluate possible organ damage. If the weapon used was contaminated, the patient is at risk of local infection, sepsis and tetanus.

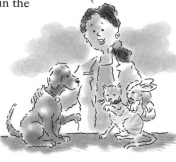

> Be aware that bites from animals, such as dogs, cats and rabbits, can cause serious infection, in addition to possible tissue damage.

Smoking gun

A gunshot wound is a high-velocity wound. Factors that affect the severity of tissue damage include the calibre of the weapon, the velocity of the projectile and the patient's position at the time of injury.

In most cases, a small-calibre weapon firing a relatively low-velocity projectile creates a small, clean punctuate lesion with little or no bleeding. If the projectile is no longer in the patient's body, treat this lesion as you would any other open wound.

A large-calibre, relatively high-velocity projectile typically causes massive tissue destruction, a large gaping wound, profuse bleeding and wound contamination. In this case, the patient requires immediate surgical intervention. After surgery, treat the wound as a surgical wound.

Assessment and care

Time is critical when caring for a patient with a traumatic wound. First, assess airway, breathing and circulation (ABC). Although focusing first on the injury itself may seem natural, a patent airway and pumping heart take priority.

Next, turn your attention to the wound. Control bleeding by applying firm, direct pressure and elevate the patient's extremities. If bleeding continues, you may need to compress a pressure point above the wound. Then assess the wound's condition. Specific wound management and cleaning depend on the type of wound and degree of contamination. (See *Caring for a patient with a traumatic wound*, page 127.)

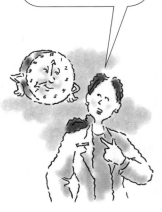

Time is critical when caring for a patient with a major traumatic wound.

Closing up

Wounds such as lacerations where tissue loss is minimal and the edges can be brought together in apposition may be closed by suture or tissue adhesive. Tissue adhesives, sometimes known as tissue glue can be used alone to close superficial wounds or in conjunction with subcutaneous sutures to close dermal wounds where deeper wound stability is necessary. They may also minimise some of the problems associated with sutures such as premature absorption or reactivity as well as improve the final cosmetic outcome. Tissue adhesives are useful for paediatric wounds where the injured child may be very anxious about having the sutures put in.

A local anaesthetic should be used prior to suturing.

Special considerations

When caring for a patient with a traumatic wound, pay particular attention to these aspects of care:
• Irrigate the wound to remove all visible contaminants from the wound bed prior to closure or dressing. This will help to decrease the risk of infection and tattooing (blue/purple scarring caused by debris remnants).
• Consider possibility of foreign bodies in the wound bed, seek specialist advice on identification (X-ray or ultrasound scan) and removal.
• Avoid using more than 8 psi of pressure when irrigating the wound. High-pressure irrigation can seriously interfere with healing by destroying cells and forcing bacteria into the tissue.
• Use sterile normal saline (0.9%) to remove debris when cleaning the wound. Alternatively, hold the injury under a running tap of potable (drinkable) water.
• Never instill hydrogen peroxide into a deep wound because the evolving gases can cause an embolism.
• Do not use alcohol to clean a traumatic wound. It's painful for the patient and dehydrates tissue.

Get wise to wounds

Caring for a patient with a traumatic wound

When treating a patient with a traumatic wound, always begin by assessing the ABC. Move on to the wound itself only after ABC is stable. Here are the basic steps to follow when caring for each type of traumatic wound.

Abrasion

- Flush the area of the abrasion with normal saline (0.9%) or potable tap water.
- Use a sterile 7.5 cm × 7.5 cm gauze pad moistened with normal saline (0.9%) to remove dirt or gravel; gently rub towards the entry point to work contaminants back out the way they entered.
- If the wound is extremely dirty, it may need to be scrubbed with a sterile surgical brush. This should be supervised by an experienced practitioner. Be as gentle as possible and keep in mind that this is a painful process for your patient.
- Allow very small wounds to dry and form a scab. Cover larger wounds with a sterile non-adherent dressing to absorb drainage and help prevent bacterial contamination.

Laceration

- Moisten a sterile 7.5 cm × 7.5 cm gauze pad with normal saline (0.9%). Gently clean the wound, beginning at the centre and working out to about 5 cm beyond the edge of the wound. Whenever the pad becomes soiled, discard it and use a new one. Continue until the wound appears clean.
- If necessary, irrigate the wound using a 50 ml catheter-tip syringe and normal saline (0.9%).
- Support the patient during wound suturing or application of adhesive wound closure strips.
- Apply a sterile non-adherent dressing over the wound to absorb drainage and help prevent bacterial contamination.

Bite

- Immediately irrigate the wound with copious amounts of normal saline (0.9%) or tap water. Do not soak the wound because this may allow bacteria to float back into the tissue.
- Clean the wound with sterile 7.5 cm × 7.5 cm gauze pads and an antiseptic solution such as povidone–iodine.
- Assist with debridement, if required.
- Apply a loose dressing. If the bite is on an extremity, elevate it to reduce swelling.
- Ask the patient about the animal that bit him to determine whether there's a risk of rabies. Administer rabies and tetanus vaccines, as needed.

Penetrating wound

- If the wound is minor, allow it to bleed for a few minutes before cleaning it. A larger puncture wound may require irrigation.
- Cover the wound with a sterile dressing.
- If the wound contains an embedded foreign object, such as a shard of glass or metal, stabilise the object until it can be removed by an experienced practitioner. When the object is removed and bleeding is under control, clean the wound as you would a laceration.
- Administer tetanus vaccine, as needed.

Whatever the cause of wound, don't forget to talk to your patient throughout the wound care procedure to reassure and calm them.

- Never use a cotton ball or a cotton-filled gauze pad to clean a wound because cotton fibres left in the wound may cause contamination or a foreign body reaction.
- If there are plans to debride the wound to remove dead tissue and reduce the risk of infection and scarring, loosely pack the wound with gauze pads soaked in normal saline (0.9%) until it's time for the procedure.
- Monitor closely for signs of developing infection, such as warm red skin or purulent discharge from the wound. Infection in a traumatic wound can delay healing, increase scarring and trigger systemic infections such as septicaemia.
- Inspect the dressing regularly. If oedema develops, adjust the dressing to ensure adequate circulation to the affected area of the wound.
- Provide analgesia as necessary and ensure your patient understands the treatment they have received and when and where to return for follow-up care.

Children and wounds

A child who is wounded, however minor the injury, is often very frightened. They may also be in pain which can be exacerbated by the fear of what might happen next. It is important, therefore, that the child and their parents are reassured about what is happening and that parental consent is gained where necessary for any procedures (such as suturing) that are required. A comforting toy, having a family member nearby and providing effective analgesia will all help to reduce the stress of the experience for the child. Dressings as such, which minimise tissue trauma and therefore pain on removal, should always be used. If dressings have adhered, soak them off with sterile normal saline (0.9%) and ask the child if they would like to help remove them. A 'well done' badge or 'just been brave' certificate is a nice reward when it's all over.

Burns

A burn is an acute wound caused by exposure to thermal extremes, electricity, caustic chemicals or radiation. The degree of tissue damage caused by a burn depends on the strength of the source and the duration of contact or exposure. Around 250 000 people per year sustain burn injuries in the UK (NBCRC 2001).

Because of the specialist care burns require, they are considered here separately from other traumatic wounds.

Types of burns

Burns can be classified by cause or type. Knowing the type of burn will help you to plan the right care for your patient.

Thermal burns

The most common type of burn, thermal burns can result from virtually any misuse or mishandling of fire, combustible products, hot fluids and fat or coming into contact with a hot object. Playing with matches, pouring petrol onto a BBQ, spilling hot coffee, touching hot hair straighteners and setting off fireworks are some common examples of ways in which burns occur. Thermal burns can also result from kitchen accidents, house or office fires, car accidents or physical abuse. Although it's less common, exposure to extreme cold can also cause thermal burns.

Electrical burns

Electrical burns result from contact with flowing electrical current. Household current, high-voltage transmission lines and lightning are sources of electrical burns. Internal injury is often considerably greater than is apparent externally.

Chemical burns

Chemical burns most commonly result from contact (skin contact or inhalation) with a caustic agent, such as an acid, an alkali or a vesicant.

Radiation burns

The most common radiation burn is sunburn, which follows excessive exposure to the sun. Almost all other burns due to radiation exposure occur as a result of radiation treatment or in specific industries that use or process radioactive materials.

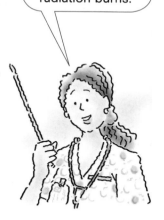

Types of burns include thermal, electrical, chemical and radiation burns.

Assessment

Conduct your initial assessment as soon as possible after the burn occurs. First, assess the patient's ABCs. Then determine the patient's level of consciousness and mobility. Next, assess the burn, including its size, depth and complexity.

Determining size

Determine burn size as part of your initial assessment. Typically, burn size is expressed as a percentage of total body surface area (TBSA). The Rule of Nines and the Lund–Browder Classification provide standardised and quick estimates of the percentage of TBSA affected. (See *Estimating burn size*, page 130.)

Estimating burn size

Several different methods can be used to estimate burn size. Because TBSA varies with age, there are differences in the methods for adult and paediatric patients.

Rule of Nines

You can quickly estimate the extent of an adult patient's burn by using the Rule of Nines. This method quantifies TBSA in multiples of 9, thus the name. To use this method, mentally transfer the burns on your patient to the body charts below. Add the corresponding percentages for each body section burned. Use the total – a rough estimate of burn extent – to calculate initial fluid replacement needs. For a child this can be modified. Up to 1 year the head is classed as 18% and each leg 14%, with the body and arms remaining the same as for adults. Then for every year after, 1% is taken off the head and ½% added to each leg. By the age of 10 years adult proportions are reached (ANZBA 2006).

Lund–Browder Classification

Although the Rule of Nines is a simple and quick way of assessing the TBSA, the use of the Lund – Browder Classification to determine burn size can be more accurate. The Lund – Browder Classification takes into account the body surface area for different ages. For example, an infant's head accounts for about 17% of their TBSA, compared with 7% for an adult.

Hands

The patient's hand equates to approximately 1%. This can be useful if estimating a small area of burn.

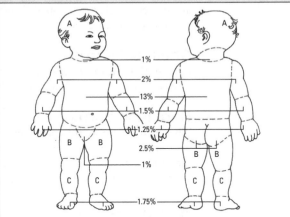

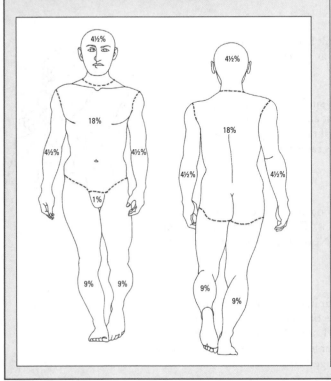

Percentage of burned body surface by age

	At birth	0 to 1 year	1 to 4 years	5 to 9 years	10 to 15 years	Adult
A: Half of head	9.5%	8.5%	6.5%	5.5%	4.5%	3.5%
B: Half of one thigh	2.75%	3.25%	4%	4.25%	4.5%	4.75%
C: Half of one leg	2.5%	2.5%	2.75%	3%	3.25%	3.5%

Memory jogger

To remember the proper sequence for the initial assessment of a burns patient, remember your ABCs and add D and E.

Airway – Assess the patient's airway, remove any obstruction and treat any obstructive condition.

Breathing – Observe the motion of the patient's chest. Auscultate the depth, rate and characteristics of the patient's breathing.

Circulation – Palpate the patient's pulse at the carotid artery and then at the distal pulse points in the wrist, posterior tibial area and foot. Loss of distal pulse may indicate shock or constriction of an extremity.

Disability – Assess the patient's level of consciousness and ability to function before attempting to move or transfer them.

Expose – Remove burned clothing from burned areas of the patient's body and thoroughly examine the skin beneath.

Determining depth

During the initial assessment, the depth of the burn needs to be determined as the depth will often have a bearing on future treatment. For example larger full thickness burns usually need surgery and skin grafting.

Four degrees of separation

The traditional method of gauging burn severity classified burn depth by degree. Today, European Guidelines (Alsbjoern 2003) suggest using depth of tissue damage to describe burns more accurately. The following method of classifying depth of burn is now commonplace:
- Superficial or epidermal burns – damage is limited to the epidermis, causing erythema and pain, no blistering. The stratum basale is unaffected. There is good capillary refill.
- Superficial partial-thickness or dermal burn – the epidermis and part of the papillary dermis are damaged, producing erythema, blisters, mild-to-moderate oedema and pain. Capillary refill will occur but the deeper the burn the slower it will be.
- Deep partial-thickness or dermal burn – the epidermis and dermis are damaged with damage extending into the reticular

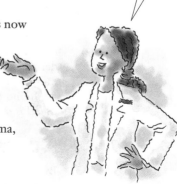

Remember, when determining burn severity, you must consider not only the size of the wound but also its depth.

Visualising burn depth

The most widely used system of classifying burn severity categorises the damage by tissue depth. However, it's important to remember that most burns involve tissue damage of varying thicknesses. This illustration may help you visualise burn damage at the various tissue depths.

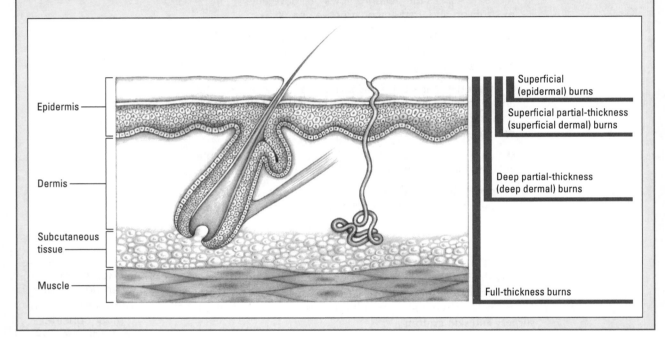

dermis; may involve sweat glands and hair follicles. The skin appears dry or moist, blotchy and red, and may be painful or painless.

Full-thickness burn – involves destruction of the epidermis and dermis and possibly subcutaneous tissue. The skin is dry and white, brown or black in colour, with no blisters. It may be described as leathery or waxy. It is painless. There is no blanching on pressure.

Full-thickness burn + involves the destruction of the epidermis, dermis, subcutaneous tissue and underlying structures such as muscle or bone.

In most instances, damage involves varying depths of injury. (See *Visualising burn depth*.)

Complex or non-complex burn?

Burns are categorised as complex or non-complex injuries. These categories take into account the degree of tissue damage and factors which will influence the care outcomes such as age, site and size of injury, mechanism of injury and coexisting medical problems (NBCRC 2001).

Complex

A burn is more likely to be complex if associated with the following:
- age under 5 or over 60 years
- dermal or full-thickness skin loss involving face, hands, perineum, feet; any flexure such as the neck; circumferential dermal or full-thickness burn of neck, torso, limb
- inhalation injury
- chemical burn >5% TBSA, suspected non-accidental injury, high tension electrical injury, ionising radiation injury, high pressure steam injury, hydrofluoric acid >1% TBSA.

The burn size will affect complexity:
- over 16 years (adult) >10% TBSA
- under 16 years (paediatric) >5% TBSA.

The presence of some coexisting conditions will also influence complexity:
- diabetes
- pregnancy
- hepatic disease
- cardiac disease or recent myocardial infarction (MI)
- immunosuppression
- respiratory disorders.

As will the presence of injuries such as fractures, crush injury, head injury and penetrating injury. All injuries that are deemed to be complex should be referred to a specialist Burns Centre or Unit.

Non-complex

Size of burn:
- over 16 years (adult), >5–10% TBSA if dermal, or smaller if full thickness
- under 16 years (paediatric), >2–5% TBSA if dermal, or smaller if full thickness
- non-complex burns should be seen in a Burns Facility or Plastic Surgery Unit.

Minor burns (those not meeting the above criteria) may be seen in an A&E or minor injuries department or in the community.

Burn care

Care for a patient with a burn depends on the type and severity of the burn, the patient's general health before the injury, and whether another injury was sustained concurrent with the burn. In general, treatment seeks to reduce pain; remove dirt, debris and dead tissue;

and provide a dressing that promotes healing. In some cases, treatment includes skin grafting.

The three FFFs

There are three main aims of burn management:
- Form – the restoration of former appearance in terms of colour, texture and contour
- Function – restoration of movement (as near as is possible) to allow daily activities to be carried out independently
- Feeling – facilitating psychological recovery.

Factors that affect healing

Factors that affect treatment and healing include:
- Burn location – burns on the face, hands, feet and genitalia are serious due to the possible loss of function
- Burn configuration – oedema due to a circumferential burn (completely encircling an extremity) can slow or stop circulation to the extremity; burns on the neck can obstruct the airway; burns on the chest can interfere with normal respiration by inhibiting expansion
- Pre-existing medical conditions – note disorders that impair peripheral circulation, especially diabetes, PVD and chronic alcohol abuse
- Other injuries sustained at the time of the burn
- Patient age – patients younger than 1 year or older than age 56 are at higher risk for complications and, consequently, for a higher mortality rate (NBCRC 2001)
- Pulmonary injury – inhaling smoke or super-heated air damages lung tissue.

First steps

First steps to take, following removal of the heat source, depend very much on the complexity or severity of the burn, a brief history if available will help to establish priorities of care quickly. Always assess the patient's ABC first. Be especially alert for signs of smoke inhalation and pulmonary damage – singed nasal hairs, mucosal burns, changes in the patient's voice, coughing, wheezing, soot in the mouth or nose or darkened sputum. If necessary, assist with endotracheal intubation and administer 100% oxygen. When the patient's ABC is stable, stop residual burning and control any bleeding.

In the case of smoke inhalation, I may need you to administer 100% oxygen.

Cool it

First remove the heat source, then apply copious amounts of water to the injured area to stop the burning process and help to relieve pain. Remove smouldering clothing, if material is stuck to the patient's skin, soak it with water or saline solution before you attempt to remove it. Remove all jewellery and any other constricting apparel.

Ideally, the water used to cool a burn should be tepid (15°C) rather than cold (never use ice). Apply to the injured area for up to 20 minutes. This will help minimise tissue damage. For small burns you can continue if it helps the pain. Care needs to be taken when cooling the burn wound, particularly with larger burns and young children, that hypothermia is not induced. This may mean restricting the length of time the burn is cooled.

Burns, apart from those on the face, can be covered with cling film initially until properly assessed. The cling film should be layered rather than wrapped around a limb to prevent the risk of constriction. Otherwise a clean (preferably sterile) sheet can be used. Remember, never cover large burns with saline-soaked dressings because this can drastically lower body temperature.

When cleaning burns, never use hydrogen peroxide or povidone–iodine (or products containing these agents) because they can cause further tissue damage and exacerbate pain considerably. Irrigating with sterile saline or showering/bathing using a mild soap such as baby bath and water will suffice.

Something to talk about

As soon as the patient's condition stabilises, and other injuries are ruled out, the patient may be given an analgesic. For severe pain, an opioid such as morphine may be necessary. Be sure to talk to the patient as you work. Emotional support and reassurance are important aspects of care and may reduce the patient's need for analgesia.

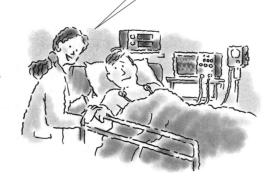

Always talk to your patient while providing burn care. Reassurance may reduce his need for analgesia.

Wrapping it up

After devitalised tissue is debrided, in theatre if necessary, cover the wound with a sterile non-adhesive, absorptive dressing; principles of moist wound healing apply as for other wounds.

Non-adherent wound contact dressings such as Urgotul™ (a hydrocolliod and petroleum mesh dressing) or Mepitel™ (a soft silicone dressing) are useful primary dressings as they can be left in place for up to 14 days. However, if the burn wound is heavily exuding then the dressing may need to be changed more frequently. If the burn wound is infected or at risk of infection a silver based dressing may be more appropriate. Foam dressings for small burns make suitable secondary dressings as they are soft, conformable and will absorb moderate amounts of exudate. In addition, hydrogels can be used to add moisture to a dry wound bed or to promote autolysis in the presence of devitalised tissue. Flamazine™ (silver sulphadiazine 1% w/w cream) should be used with caution (see Cochrane Reviews website, page 275), as it may delay healing. If using, do not apply until the burn wound has been expertly assessed as it will mask the true depth of the burn. There are many potentially suitable dressings available; if you are unsure it is advisable to contact your local burns service for advice.

Keep on with it

Secure the dressings, taking care to minimise the risk of skin trauma or vessel/limb constriction. Elastic netting or crepe bandages loosely applied are ideal for this purpose as they expand to accommodate the swelling associated with oedema and are frequently seen following burns injuries.

Blister busters

Blisters occur when the epidermal and dermal layers are separated by heat and fluid fills the empty space. Blisters are not all treated in the same way. Small blisters can be left intact where possible to minimise the risk of infection. For larger blisters, those that are likely to burst and those that compromise function because of where they are situated, opinion is divided as to whether, using an aseptic technique, they should be debrided or aspirated using a fine needle. It is recommended that you follow the advice and guidelines of your local burn service. Remember, only experienced personnel should perform debridement or aspiration.

For further advice on the management of epidermal and dermal burns please see page 275 for the relevant NHS Clinical Knowledge Summary website.

Solution resolution

A patient with serious burns needs massive fluid replacement – especially during the first 24 hours after the injury. Begin intravenous (I.V.) therapy, as ordered, to prevent hypovolaemic shock and help maintain cardiac output.

What goes in must come out

Closely monitor the patient's intake and output and check vital signs often. If the patient's limbs are badly burned, measuring blood pressure may be difficult; in this instance follow local procedure for obtaining a blood pressure measurement. Finally, be prepared to assist in emergency escharotomy if the patient's burns threaten circulation of the limbs.

Electrical burns

Tissue damage from electrical burns is difficult to assess because internal damage along the conduction pathway is commonly greater than the surface burn indicates. If possible, determine the voltage involved. This information helps the healthcare team assess possible internal damage more accurately.

Keep in mind that current passing through the body can induce ventricular fibrillation, cardiac arrest or respiratory arrest – all life-threatening conditions requiring immediate intervention. (See *Electric shock*.)

Chemical burns

When treating a patient who has a chemical burn, begin by irrigating the wound with copious amounts of water for 20 minutes or more. Take care that the water, which will have become contaminated with the chemical following irrigation, does not come into contact with you or collect around the patient to avoid the risk of further chemical burns. Alkalis usually produce more severe burns than acids; however, the severity of the burn is usually determined by the length of time that the chemical was in contact with the patient's skin.

Electric shock

When electric current passes through the body, the damage it does depends on:

- intensity of the current (measured in amperes)
- resistance of the tissues it passes through
- kind of current (alternating current, direct current or a combination of both)
- frequency and duration of the current's flow.

Electric current can cause injury in three ways:

- true electrical injury caused by current that passes through the body
- arc or flash burns caused by current that doesn't pass through the body
- thermal surface burns caused by associated heat and flames.

The patient's prognosis depends on:

- site of the injury
- extent of damage
- his general health prior to the injury
- speed and adequacy of treatment.

If the patient's eyes are involved, flush them with plenty of water or saline solution for at least 30 minutes. If it's an alkaline burn, irrigate until the pH of the cul-de-sacs returns to 7.0. Then have the patient close their eyes and cover them with sterile dressings. Arrange for an ophthalmological examination. Finally, note the type of chemical involved and the presence of any noxious fumes.

Special considerations

Consider the following when caring for a patient with a burn:
• Assess the patient's level of pain, including non-verbal indications, and administer analgesics, such as morphine intravenously, as prescribed. (Avoid intramuscular injections because tissue damage associated with the burn injury may impair drug absorption.)
• Keep the patient calm, provide periods of uninterrupted rest between procedures, and use non-pharmacological pain relief measures, as appropriate.
• Prepare the patient for possible grafting, as indicated.

Potential complications

Potential complications that may arise include:
• hypovolaemic shock
• fluid overload
• pulmonary oedema
• infection.
  Be sure to monitor the patient's vital signs and haemodynamic parameters and assess for signs and symptoms of infection, such as fever, elevated WBC count and changes in burn wound appearance or drainage.

Follow-up

Burns patients will often need prolonged multi-professional support to ensure optimum form, function and feeling is achieved. Many other specialists will work alongside the medical and nursing staff to support the patient through post-injury period. For example:
• physiotherapists
• occupational therapists
• dietitians
• prosthetic limb-fitters
• pyschologists
• surgical appliance technicians
• pharmacists
• skin camouflage technicians.

Skin grafting

Skin grafting may be necessary to repair defects caused by burns, trauma or surgery. Depending on the graft's complexity, the procedure is usually performed under local or general anaesthesia and, in some cases, may be performed as an outpatient procedure. (For information on temporary skin grafts, see *Biological dressings*, page 85.)

The surgeon may choose skin grafting as the preferred treatment option if:
- primary closure isn't possible or cosmetically acceptable
- primary closure would interfere with function
- there is extensive skin loss
- reconstructive surgery is required following trauma or removal of malignant tissue
- a skin tumour is excised and the site needs to be monitored for recurrence.

Three types of skin grafts exist:
- split-thickness grafts – consisting of the epidermis and a small portion of the dermis
- full-thickness grafts – consisting of the epidermis and all of the dermis
- composite grafts – consisting of the epidermis, dermis and underlying tissues (such as muscle, cartilage and bone).

Secret of success

The success or failure of any skin graft depends on revascularisation. Initially, a skin graft survives by direct contact with the underlying tissue, receiving oxygen and nutrients through existing blood vessels. However, the graft will die unless new blood vessels develop. For split-thickness grafts, revascularisation usually takes 3 to 5 days; for full-thickness grafts, it may take up to 2 weeks.

Fall harvest

The graft is taken, or harvested, from an area of healthy tissue on the patient's body. Therefore, it's important to provide meticulous skin care to preserve potential donor sites. Also, because graft survival depends on close contact with underlying tissue, the recipient site – the wound – should be healthy granulation tissue that's free from eschar, debris and infection. If the skin is taken from the patient themselves, it may also be referred to as an allograft.

The donor site of a split thickness graft can often be more painful than the grafted area itself, so appropriate analgesia is required. If appropriate, the dressing is left on the donor site for up

Cover for success

Skin substitutes

The ideal covering to achieve healing for a full-thickness burn wound is a skin graft harvested from the patient's own undamaged skin. However, in some situations this is not possible, or where the burn is only partial thickness a skin substitute or biological dressing may be used. Biological dressings function much like skin grafts, preventing infection and fluid loss and easing patient discomfort. However, biological dressings are only temporary measures because the body eventually rejects them. If the underlying wound hasn't healed, the dressing must be replaced with a graft of the patient's own skin.

Here's a comparison of autografts with five types of biological dressings that can be used as a skin substitute.

Type and source	Use and duration	Special considerations
Autograft Graft from one part of body to another in the same person	• Used to cover tissue loss. If wound bed is clean and infection-free, it should take permanently	• Observe the wound for exudate. Avoid shearing to the graft and build-up of haematomas and seromas. • Watch for local signs of infection or graft failure.
Allograft (homograft) Grafted from one individual to another in the same species. Usually harvested from cadavers	• Used to protect excisions and to temporarily cover burns when the patient doesn't have sufficient skin for immediate grafting. Also used to cover meshed grafts, to protect exposed tendons. • Usually rejected in 7 to 10 days	• Observe the wound for exudate. • Watch for local and systemic signs of rejection.
Amnion Made from amnion and chorionic membranes	• Used to protect burns and to temporarily cover granulation tissue awaiting a graft • Must be changed every 48 hours	• Apply only to clean wounds. • Cover with a dressing.
Biosynthetic Woven from man-made fibres	• Used to cover donor sites and partial-thickness burns; to protect clean, superficial burns and excised wounds awaiting grafts • If applied to a partial-thickness wound, it is usually left in place untill it heals underneath and peals off easily	• Apply only to clean wounds. • Don't remove to treat the wound (biosynthetic dressings are permeable to antimicrobials).
Cultured skin cells Skin cells culture from a biopsy taken from the patients healthy skin	• Used with widely meshed skin grafts and on donor sites to speed up wound healing and coverage	• Cover with a dressing. • Avoid shearing.
Xenograft (heterograft) Grafted from one animal to another. Usually harvested from pigs	• Used for same purposes as an allograft • Usually rejected in 7 to 10 days	• Cover with a dressing. • Watch for signs of rejection.

to 10 days so as to avoid disturbing the epithealisation process. Full thickness grafts are often taken from an area that has some surplus skin so that direct closure of the donor area can be achieved, such as the groin or postauricular. The suture line then needs to be kept clean and observed for infection.

Survival of the fittest

After a patient receives a skin graft, all aspects of care focus on promoting graft survival. Help the patient find comfortable positions for relaxing and sleeping that prevent him from lying on the area of the graft. If feasible, keep the graft elevated and immobilised. When needed, modify your routine to accommodate healing and prevent shearing of the graft. For example, never use a blood pressure cuff over a graft site. Administer analgesics as necessary; however, remember to teach the patient techniques to reduce pain that don't involve medication (such as relaxation techniques).

The first graft dressing may be changed between 3–7 days depending on where it is. Always use sterile technique when changing dressings and work gently to avoid dislodging the graft. Aspirate any serous pockets or haematomas. Clean the graft site with warm (from a thermostatically controlled warming cabinet) normal saline (0.9%) Often a non-adherent dressing such as Mepitel™ is used, however if a fine-mesh gauze has been placed over the graft this can be left intact for several days. Then cover the area with gauze and a crepe bandage.

There's no place like home

As the patient prepares to go home, discuss proper care with them. Explain that the dressings on the graft and donor sites shouldn't be disturbed for any reason. If they feel the dressing needs to be changed, they should contact the ward for advice and never attempt to do it themselves. Emphasise that immobilising the area of the graft is essential for speedy and complete healing. Later, as healing progresses, they can apply moisturiser to the graft site several times a day to keep the skin pliable and help the scar mature. In some cases, pressure garments may also be required to promote a better appearance of the scar.

Sun exposure can affect graft pigmentation. Explain this to the patient and suggest that they limit the amount of time they spend in the sun. Also suggest that they use UV sunblock anytime they plan to be outdoors.

Finally, almost all patients express concern about scarring and appearance. Explain that if scarring continues to be a problem when the graft completely heals, there may be plastic surgery options which will help.

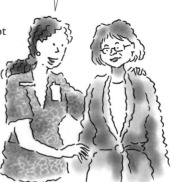

Be sure to teach your patient not to disturb the dressing on their graft and donor sites after they are discharged home.

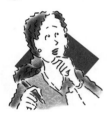

Quick quiz

1.   After abdominal surgery, your patient says that they felt something 'pop' when they were getting back into bed. You examine their wound and find bowel protruding. You should:

    A.   place the patient in high Fowler's position
    B.   place the patient in low Fowler's position
    C.   place the patient flat in bed
    D.   place the patient on their left side.

Answer: B. Place the patient in low Fowler's position to reduce tension on the wound.

2.   What's the first step in caring for a patient with a traumatic wound?

    A.   get them to the hospital
    B.   take a blood pressure measurement
    C.   apply pressure bandages
    D.   assess their airway, breathing and circulation.

Answer: D. Your first priority is to assess the patient's airway, breathing and circulation.

3.   When assessing your patient's burns, you note damage to the epidermis, dermis and subcutaneous tissue. What type of burn have they suffered?

    A.   superficial partial-thickness dermal
    B.   deep partial-thickness dermal
    C.   full-thickness
    D.   full-thickness +

Answer: C. In a full-thickness burn, the epidermis, dermis and subcutaneous tissue are damaged.

4.   Your patient has deep partial-thickness and full-thickness burn injuries to the posterior portion of both legs as well as their entire left and right arms. Using the Rule of Nines, what percentage of TBSA is involved?

    A.   18%
    B.   27%
    C.   36%
    D.   45%

Answer: C. The posterior portion of both legs constitutes 18% of TBSA and the entire left and right arms constitute another 18%, for a total of 36%.

5. Which intervention can best protect the skin around a heavily draining surgical incision from irritation due to wound drainage?
    A. applying a wound drainage bag (pouching) to the wound
    B. applying packing and gauze dressings
    C. applying a hydrocolloid dressing
    D. applying an occlusive dressing.

Answer: A. Applying a wound drainage bag prevents irritation of surrounding tissue when there's copious drainage from an incision.

6. To prevent skin tears, you should:
    A. encourage the patient to wear short-sleeve tops
    B. use adhesive tape on dressings
    C. tell the patient to avoid sudden movements
    D. avoid using skin lotion.

Answer: C. Encourage your patient to avoid sudden or brusque movements that can pull the skin and possibly cause a skin tear.

7. Your patient has a surgical wound that has been closed for 8 days. During your wound assessment, you palpate a ridge along the incision line. This ridge may indicate:
    A. normal healing
    B. wound dehiscence
    C. wound evisceration
    D. wound tunnelling.

Answer: A. This ridge, known as the healing ridge, is a sign that normal healing is progressing.

Scoring

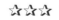 If you answered all seven questions correctly, strut your stuff! You've demonstrated an acute understanding of the chapter.

If you answered five or six questions correctly, you deserve a hand! Your surgical approach to studying has served you well.

If you answered fewer than five questions correctly, that's okay! After a quick review, you'll be healed in no time.

References

Ahn, C., Mulligan, P. and Salcido, R.S. (2008) Smoking – the bane of wound healing: biomedical interventions and social influences. *Advances in Skin and Wound Care* 12(5):227–236.

Alsbjoern, B.F. (2003) *European Practice guidelines for Burn Care.* Copenhagen EBA meeting, September 2002.

Australian and New Zealand Burn Association education committee. (2006) *Emergency Management of Severe Burns Manual.* 10th edn. Australian and New Zealand Burn Association

Benbow, M. (2005) *Evidence-based Wound Management.* London: Whurr.

Bryant, R. and Nix, D. (2006) *Acute and Chronic Wounds: Nursing Management.* 3rd edn. St.Louis: Mosby.

Horan, T.C., Gaynes, R.P., Martone, W.J. *et al.* (1992) CDC definitions of nosocomial surgical site infections, 1992: a modification of CDC definitions of surgical wound infections. *Infection Control and Hospital Epidemiology* 13:606–608.

Linblad, W.J. (1998) Tensile strength of a wound: its use in human wound healing studies. *Wound Repair and Regeneration* 6(2):178–179.

Lock, P.M. (1979) The effects of temperature on mitotic activity at the edge of experimental wounds. In Sundell, B. (ed) *Wound Healing Plastic, Surgical and Dermatological Aspects. Symposium – Papers and Discussion,* pp. 103–109. Finland: ESPOO.

Myers, B.A. (2004) *Wound Management Principles.* New Jersey: Prentice Hall.

National Burns Care Review Committee (NBCRC) (2001) *Standards and Strategy for Burn Care – A Review of Burn Care in the British Isles.* London: NBCRC.

National Institute of Health and Clinical Excellence (NICE) (2008) *CG74 Surgical Site Infection: Prevention and Treatment of Surgical Site Infection.* London: RCOG Press.

Payne, R.L. and Martin, M.L. (1993) Defining and classifying skin tears: need for a common language. *Ostomy Wound Managment* 39(5):16–20, 22–24, 26.

Smyth, E. (2006) *Late Breaker – Preliminary results of third national prevalence survey of healthcare-associated infections.* Sixth International Conference of the Hospital Infection Society, Amsterdam. (18 October 2006).

Smyth, E.T., McIlvenny, G., Enstone, J.E. *et al.* (2008) Four country healthcare associated infection prevalence survey 2006: overview of the results. *Journal of Hospital Infection* 69(3):230–248.

Wienert, P., Heiss, J., Rinecker, H. and Sing, A. (1999) A human bite. *Lancet* 354(9178):572.

7 Non-healing wounds

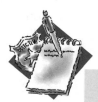

Just the facts

In this chapter, you'll learn:

♦ causes of non-healing wounds
♦ the role of wound bed preparation
♦ assessment of non-healing wounds
♦ management of non-healing wounds
♦ important teaching points for patients and their carers.

A look at non-healing wounds

A non-healing (chronic) wound is typically defined as a wound that fails to follow the normal healing process.

Wound bed preparation

Wound bed preparation is a framework that can be used to manage the critical components of a non-healing wound in a structured way (Dowsett 2008). In other words, it helps the healthcare practitioner to think about the key elements of the wound that are causing problems and to find the right solutions to move the wound towards healing again. In a non-healing wound there are often multiple reasons why the wound is failing to progress. The patient, their history and their wound must be assessed carefully to elicit these reasons.

Causes

Common causes of non-healing wounds include infection and inadequate wound bed perfusion and oxygenation. Non-healing wounds can also result from malignancy and chronic disease

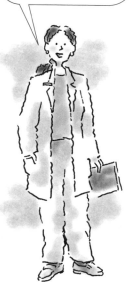

When all standard approaches to wound healing fail, the wound becomes chronic and is classified as non-healing.

processes such as diabetes. Some wounds are caused by the patient themselves and some fail to heal because of patient interference, these are called factitious wounds. Hypergranulation tissue (proud flesh) in the wound bed may also result in delays or non-healing.

Infection

Non-healing wounds may be infected with a range of bacteria including *Klebsiella, Proteus, Pseudomonas, Staphylococcus, Clostridium* and *Bacteroides fragilis*. Typically, these infected wounds don't show the classic signs of infection, such as oedema, redness and purulent drainage. In some instances, prolonged inflammation; discoloured or bleeding, friable granulation tissue; pocketing at the base of the wound; and the absence of healing may be the only signs of infection.

Detective work

If an infection remains undetected, the wound won't heal. This can lead to amputation and other serious complications such as osteomyelitis. When a wound fails to heal, suspect infection and evaluate the wound accordingly. Do remember that some non-healing wounds are related to systemic rather than local infection, for example, the sexually transmitted disease syphilis causes chancres (small, painless ulcers) to form at the point of bacterial entry e.g. around the anus, mouth, vagina and penis.

Immune disorders

Reduced immunity will increase the risk of opportunistic bacteria entering open wounds and of fungal infections such as candidiasis (thrush) taking hold. Disorders of the immune system such as late-stage/advanced HIV infection (also referred to as acquired immunodeficiency syndrome (AIDS)) can affect the skin in a variety of ways including the development of multiple skin lesions associated with Kaposi's sarcoma (a type of cancer – see *Malignancy*, page 147).

Poor perfusion

Inadequate perfusion or oxygenation impairs healing and increases the risk of infection. Inadequate perfusion can result from underlying disorders such as peripheral vascular disease which lead to a reduced quantity of blood in the peripheral vascular system. Insufficient oxygenation can result from disorders like anaemia or chronic respiratory disorders such as obstructive airways disease, both of these result in a reduction of circulating oxygen.

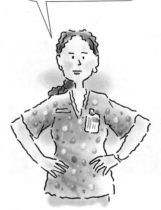

Infection, malignancy and inadequate perfusion can cause non-healing wounds.

Malignancy

Patients can also develop non-healing wounds as a result of a primary or secondary malignancy. About 5% to 20% of patients with metatastic (spreading) cancer will develop non-healing, malignant cutaneous wounds (Haisfield-Wolfe and Rund 1997). Some cancers may ulcerate as they outgrow their blood supply, and some chronic wounds have been known to develop into squamous cell carcinomas. A non-healing, malignant wound may appear at the site of malignant disease or at a site distal to the malignancy. These types of wounds are most commonly associated with breast cancer but they can also occur from other malignancies, such as cancer of the head, neck, chest, abdomen, kidney, lung, ovary, colon and penis as well as from leukaemia, lymphoma and melanoma.

Disorganisation dilemma

Cancer cells are typically disorganised with poorly differentiated borders as a result of the malignant change that alters their normal behaviour. When a cell becomes cancerous, it begins to rob surrounding tissues of oxygen and nutrients. Malignant cells begin to secrete tissue permeability factor, which increases vascular permeability. This leads to increased production of exudate, which causes loss of protein and fibrinogen. Thus, malignant wounds are prone to bleeding because they're highly vascular and have poor clotting tendencies.

Breaking down

Bacterial proteases (enzymes present in necrotic tissue) cause the breakdown of tissue. Malignant wounds tend to have a large amount of necrotic tissue because they fail to heal; therefore, they also have an increased number of bacterial proteases present. With the presence of non-viable, necrotic tissue and excessive exudate, malignant wounds provide an ideal medium for aerobic and anaerobic organism growth, which can cause these wounds to have a foul odour. Aerobic bacteria that may cause odour include *Klebsiella*, *Proteus*, *Pseudomonas* and *Staphylococcus*. Anaerobic bacteria that may cause odour include *Clostridium* and *Bacteroides fragilis*.

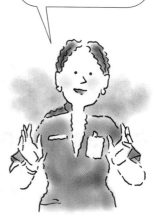

Aerobic and anaerobic organisms commonly grow in malignant wounds, causing a foul odour.

Size reducers

Chemotherapy and radiation treatments can reduce the size of a malignant wound. The smaller wound may become more manageable in terms of wound drainage, odour and bleeding. However, chemotherapy and radiation may also cause peri-wound (skin around the wound) irritation, which may lead to further wound breakdown. Wounds can also develop if chemotherapy drugs leak into the tissues. In addition, some cytoxic drugs are irritants and will cause pain or inflammation without necrosis, while other drugs, such as vesicants, can cause severe pain and may result in severe tissue damage.

Factitious wounds

Self inflicted (self harm) or factitious wounds are hard to diagnose and difficult to treat. The factitious wound often presents atypically and the patient history may be incongruent with the clinical presentation. Elimination of other causes of failure to heal, combined with a detailed patient history, will help towards diagnosis, whilst a sensitively taken history may reveal the underlying reason for self harming. Understanding the reasons behind factitious wounding is key to getting the right patient support and treatment. For clinical guidance on managing self-harming patients (CG16 Self Harm) see the NICE website, page 275.

Hypergranulating wounds

Hypergranulation (proud flesh) is an excess of granulation tissue beyond the amount required to replace the tissue deficit incurred as a result of skin injury or wounding. It can delay wound closure and adversely affect the wound's final appearance. The exact cause is unknown but it has been linked to chronic inflammation, wound hypoxia and high bacterial burden. Different management approaches are needed for different causes. Malignancy should always be ruled out before proceeding with treatment.

Assessment

When assessing a patient with a non-healing wound, the T.I.M.E. assessment framework can be used to put wound bed preparation into practice by focusing attention on the critical components of a non-healing wound. T.I.M.E. is an acronym which stands for:

T – tissue management
I – control of inflammation or infection
M – moisture balance
E – advancement of the epithelial edge of the wound

(See *Using the T.I.M.E. framework*.)

In addition to assessing the critical components of the non-healing wound, it is important to obtain a thorough patient history and examine the wound carefully.

Using the T.I.M.E. framework

The T.I.M.E. framework focuses on the removal of non-viable tissue such as slough or necrotic tissue (tissue management), ensuring the wound is neither too wet nor too dry (moisture balance), the reduction of inflammation and resolution of infection (control of inflammation and infection) and the advancement of new epidermal cells from the wound edge across the surface of the wound (advancement of epithelial edge). When these issues have been adressed, the wound bed should be well prepared for healing.

History

If you suspect a non-healing wound, you need to gather information about the wound's development. Remember to ask the patient these questions:

- When did the wound develop? What was the cause?
- What wound treatments have you undergone (if any)?
- When was your last chemotherapy or radiation treatment (if applicable)?
- Has the appearance of the wound changed? If so, how?
- Has the wound exudate changed in colour, amount or odour?

Then assess the patient's medication history, the presence of diseases and their nutritional status.

Medications

Certain medications may influence wound healing. Keep in mind that medications such as steroids, antivirals, antibiotics and antineoplastics can be immunosuppressive, affecting the body's ability to respond to a wound infection. Herbal and other non-traditional medications can also influence the patient's risk of infection. When you obtain a medication history, remember to ask if the patient has used or is using any non-traditional medications.

Diseases

The presence of more than one disease may also increase the patient's risk for infection. Be particularly alert to diseases that impact on the vascular, pulmonary and immune systems. Diseases, such as cancer, autoimmune disorders and AIDS, can impact on the body's ability to respond to infection and can alter the appearance of an infected wound. If the patient's immune system is compromised, an infected wound may fail to exhibit the classic signs of infection.

Cancer connection

Question the patient carefully (and sensitively) about any history of cancer, including the type of cancer and any metastasis to other sites. Remember that certain cancers are more likely to cause non-healing wounds. Cancers of the head, neck, chest/breast and abdomen are most commonly related to malignant wounds.

Radiation ramifications

Treatment for cancer usually includes chemotherapy and radiation. Chemotherapy drugs can cause adverse effects as immunosuppression, GI disturbances and mucous membrane ulceration. GI disturbances, such as chronic diarrhoea, can lead to excoriated skin, which can predispose the patient to infection and wound development.

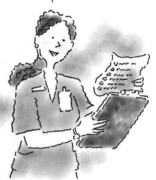

When obtaining a patient history, be sure to ask the patient when their wound developed and ask about any past or current treatments, including medications they may be taking.

Immunosuppression can affect the body's ability to fight infection. In turn, ulceration of mucous membranes may cause wound development in an immunocompromised patient. Ask the patient when they last received chemotherapy and if they experienced adverse effects.

Radiation therapy can also contribute to the development of non-healing wounds. If the patient is undergoing radiation treatment, determine the type of radiation and how many treatments have been administered and identify adverse effects the patient has experienced.

Radiation-induced skin damage can appear in different ways:
- mild erythema and oedema similar to a sunburn
- dry desquamation characterised by hyperpigmented, intact skin that's dry, itching, peeling and flaking
- moist desquamation characterised by exposure of the dermis with peeling, blistering and exudate
- deep dermal damage characterised by ulcerations and necrosis; hair follicles and sweat or sebaceous glands may also be injured.

Additionally, radiation recall (a severe skin reaction) can occur in the field of treatment when chemotherapy is given concurrently or subsequent to radiation therapy with skin damage that occurs several weeks after the radiation has ended.

Nutritional status

The patient's nutritional status can influence the development of a non-healing wound and whether it will eventually heal. Evaluate the patient's diet to determine if he's consuming enough calories and protein to promote wound healing. Obtaining blood tests such as albumin and electrolyte levels, can also provide important information about the patient's nutritional status.

If you discover that the patient is malnourished, try to find the cause. The patient may fail to consume enough calories for various reasons, including lack of money, disliking the taste of the food or poor appetite. All of these factors must be considered when discussing a nutritional plan with the patient. Keep in mind that cultural influences can also impact concordance with an ordered diet.

> Poor nutrition can influence the development of a non-healing wound. Be sure to evaluate your patient's diet to determine if he's consuming enough calories and protein.

Psychosocial effects

Non-healing wounds are often accompanied by one or more distressing symptoms; these can impact significantly on the patient's quality of life. Excessive wound exudate, bleeding and odour may lead the patient to isolate themselves from their family and social situations rather than risk embarrassment. In addition, altered body image and lowered self-esteem can cause the patient to feel less attractive to their partner. Also, many partners become carers, performing wound care and hygiene for the patient. This may cause the relationship between the patient and their partner to become more like a patient–carer relationship rather than an intimate one.

Pain can also be problematic, chronic pain can result in appetite loss, sleep disturbances and depression as well as feelings of anger and guilt. Communication may be affected and family and carers may feel shut out and helpless.

The impact of a non-healing wound on family, work and social life should not be underestimated. Listen carefully to your patients concerns and endeavour to minimise the psychosocial impact of their wound through appropriate treatment selection and the provision of ongoing support and encouragement to the whole family.

Physical examination

Assess a wound that fails to follow the normal healing process for infection. To determine the presence of an infection, evaluate the patient's wound for evidence of local and systemic infection and bone involvement. The wound may have non-viable or hypergranulating tissue and may demonstrate delays in epithelial migration leading to wound closure. Remember, in addition to assessing the wound, you should always perform a thorough physical examination, including vital signs.

Evidence of infection

Some wounds may demonstrate clear signs of infection, including erythema, oedema, purulent drainage, unexpected or increased pain and foul odour. Systemic signs of infection include cellulitis extending at least 1 cm beyond the wound margin, fever, elevated WBC count and high blood glucose levels. However, some wounds may fail to demonstrate the obvious signs of infection; therefore, you must carefully consider the patient history as well as the wound in order to determine if infection is likely. (See *Recognising infection*, page 40.)

Perform a wound culture and sensitivity only if clinical indicators suggest it is necessary. (See *Wound specimen collection*, page 77.)

Behind the mask

Signs of infection in patients with diabetes or arterial disease may be subtle or masked. In some cases, inflammation that persists longer than 5 days; discoloration of the wound bed; bleeding, friable granulation tissue; the presence of pocketing at the base of the wound; and the absence of healing may indicate infection.

Unwelcome guest

Examine the wound's appearance. Malignant wounds have been described as rapidly growing (like a fungus) and cauliflower-like in appearance. You may also find that the patient's wound has non-viable tissue and may bleed easily because malignant wounds tend to have poor perfusion and reduced clotting tendencies. Carefully assess the malignant wound for the presence of sinus tracts or fistulas because malignant cells tend to invade surrounding tissues and organs.

As malignant cells invade the surrounding tissue, pruritus (itching) may develop due to stretching of the skin and irritation of peripheral nerve fibres. Fungal infections may also cause pruritus. Evaluate for pruritus and be sure to ask the patient about products he's using to alleviate the itching. Antihistamines typically have no effect on the pruritus that's associated with malignant wounds.

Wet, wet, wet

Both malignant and infected wounds often produce copious amounts of exudate. These wounds may also have a foul odour. Estimate the amount of wound exudate and assess its colour, consistency and odour. You should also evaluate the peri-wound for maceration caused by excess exudate and for excoriation caused by the destructive enzymes contained in chronic wound exudate (called matrix metalloproteinases). Maceration is seen as a spongy, delicate tissue which is whitish in colour. Excoriation is seen as reddened, inflamed skin, superficially broken, sometimes bleeding and often very sore/painful.

Bone involvement

An X-ray of the affected area can't be relied on to help determine bone involvement because it can take 10 to 21 days for bone changes to be visible on an X-ray. A bone biopsy is considered the gold standard when diagnosing osteomyelitis; however, because it's invasive, non-invasive tests, such as a bone scan or MRI, are often preferred.

Suspect osteomyelitis in any non-healing wound that probes to the bone. Osteomyelitis is a serious complication in which bacterial organisms have invaded the bone tissue. It commonly leads to removal of the infected bone or amputation of the affected extremity.

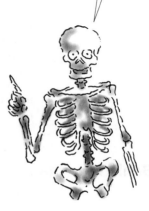

Non-invasive tests, such as a bone scan or MRI, are preferred when diagnosing osteomyelitis.

Diagnostic tests

Diagnostic tests that can be performed to determine if a wound is non-healing include:

- WBC and differential count – used to obtain information about the presence and type of infection and whether the infection is acute or chronic. (It can also help evaluate the patient's immune system function which, if compromised, can lead to an increased risk for bleeding and poor tissue perfusion.)
- Red blood cell and platelet count – used to evaluate the patient's immune function as a result of treatment with chemotherapy and radiation; a low count may indicate an increased risk for bleeding and poor tissue perfusion.
- Tissue biopsy – used to confirm the diagnosis of a malignant wound; particularly important if the wound developed without any known cause.
- MRI and computerised tomography and bone scans – used to obtain information regarding the metastasis of cancer and which organs and tissues the cancer has infiltrated (these tests also provide information about bone involvement and help diagnose osteomyelitis).
- Wound culture and sensitivity – used to determine the number and specific type of aerobic and anaerobic bacteria, which can also help determine appropriate antibiotic therapy.

Treatment

After thorough assessment, refer back to the T.I.M.E. framework to determine which key factors are impacting on wound healing and how they can be eliminated or managed. Remember also to consider the management of exudate, odour and pain which are often the most distressing aspects of having a wound. With non-healing wounds caused by an end stage malignancy, the goals of treatment should be based on symptom control and comfort, rather than healing.

The goals of treating non-healing, malignant wounds are symptom control and comfort.

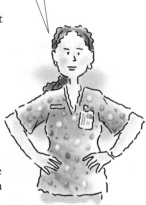

Controlling exudate

Controlling exudate is one of the primary goals of non-healing wound management. Several dressing options are available, including calcium alginate, foam and hydrofibre dressings, which provide good absorption in wounds with moderate-to-large amounts of exudate. The use of wound drainage systems, such as pouches or suction systems, can also be an effective option for wounds with large amounts of exudate.

A word of caution

Keep in mind that dressings may cause trauma and bleeding if they become adhered to the wound bed. This can happen as exudate levels diminish and dressings dry out.

Controlling odour

Dressings that contain charcoal, such as CarboFlex® or charcoal and silver such as Actisorb Plus®, help to control wound odour as do honey-based dressings such as Mesitran®.

Frequent dressing changes and careful attention to hygiene can also aid in odour control. The topical application of metronidazole (Metrotop®) has been reported to decrease and control odour in fungating wounds (Paul and Pieper 2008).

Controlling pain

Pain can be an important issue in non-healing wounds. Be sure to assess the patient for pain by using a reliable and valid pain assessment tool, such as the visual analog, numeric pain intensity or FACES pain rating scales, and make sure that appropriate pain management techniques are implemented. (For further information refer to the World Union of Wound Healing Societies consensus document (2004) – *Minimising pain at wound dressing related procedures*.) Premedication before dressing changes can increase the patient's comfort. Analgesics may be prescribed according to the World Health Organization's Pain Ladder (WHO 2008) adapted for use in wound pain by Senecal (1999). The use of self-administered oxygen and nitrous oxide gas (Entonox®) may also be considered for short-term pain relief during an uncomfortable or painful wound related procedure.

Topical solution

In addition, topical anaesthetics may reduce the amount of pain experienced by the patient during dressing changes and throughout the day. Topical application of medications, such as EMLA (lidocaine and prilocaine) cream have been found to be effective in reducing the pain associated with debridement in venous leg ulceration (Briggs and Nelson 2001), however, EMLA is not currently licensed for use in the UK. When assessing the evidence base for any intervention it is always important to consider the context in which the product will be used.

Complementary therapies, such as massage and aromatherapy, and self-help techniques such as visulisation, may also help the patient with pain control.

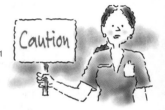

Be careful when using a calcium alginate dressing for a bleeding wound with minimal exudate because the dressing may adhere to the wound bed and damage tissue.

Controlling bleeding

In some non-healing wounds, particularly malignant wounds, bleeding is an issue. Non-adherent dressings should be utilised to reduce trauma to the wound tissue and reduce the risk of bleeding. Contact layers made of soft silicone will prevent outer dressings from sticking to the wound bed. Other appropriate dressings for a bleeding wound include calcium alginates and hydrofibres. In addition, some dressings, such as calcium alginate may encourage coagulation (Segal *et al.* 1998). (See *Dressings used for non-healing wounds.*) Keep in mind that calcium alginate dressings are indicated for wounds with heavy drainage and should be used with caution in bleeding wounds with minimal exudate because they could adhere to the wound bed and damage tissue when removed.

Dress for success

Dressings used for non-healing wounds

Use this chart to help you determine which dressing or medication to use on a non-healing wound.

Wound characteristics	Dressings	Medications
Exudate	• Foam • Alginate • Hydrofibre	• Topical antimicrobial dressings (silver or iodine-based) if wound infection present
Odour	• Foam • Alginate • Hydrofibre • Charcoal • Honey	• Topical metronidazole • Topical antimicrobial dressings (silver or iodine-based) if wound infection present
Pain	• Silicone • Hydrogel (if wound has minimal drainage) • Foam • Alginate • Hydrofibre	• Topical anaesthetics • Oral or parenteral pain medications • Topical analgesia
Bleeding	• Alginate • Hydrofibre • Gelatin-based haemostatic (such as Gelfoam® or Spongostan®)	• Topical adrenaline (use with caution)

Adrenaline rush

Topical adrenaline, which causes local vasoconstriction, is sometimes used to control bleeding, however, this vasoconstriction can lead to poor tissue perfusion. Topical adrenalin should be used with caution and only by a member of the medical team.

Managing infection

Topical antimicrobial dressings such as those containing silver, iodine or honey, can effectively reduce the bacterial burden of the wound and resolve distressing local symptoms such as excess exudate, odour and pain. Removal of non-viable tissue where possible will also reduce wound bioburden.

Debridement removal of non-viable tissue

Wound debridement and cleaning are effective measures to reduce the amount of non-viable tissue and the bacterial load in a wound. Several options are available, including autolysis, enzymatic, surgical, conservative sharp debridement and biological (larvae) therapy.

The decision to use a specific method of debridement depends on several factors, such as:
- cause or source of the wound
- location of the wound
- extent of infection
- amount and extent of necrosis
- type of tissue
- healing potential
- risk for bleeding and pain
- comorbidity factors
- the patient's and family's wishes.

Surgical and sharp (scalpel or scissors) debridement must only be carried out by a qualified healthcare professional trained to perform the procedure safely and competently. (See Chapter 3, *Basic Wound Care Procedures*.)

Weighing the benefits

You should weigh the benefits of debridement against the risk of exposing the protected surface of a wound when healing may be delayed or isn't expected. In patients with non-healing wounds related to poor tissue perfusion with no chance of tissue revascularisation, debridement of the protective eschar can lead to further complications and should be avoided.

Think nutrition

Clean plate please . . .

Remember, the patient with a non-healing wound needs to increase his consumption of protein because a non-healing wound tends to produce excessive exudate, which leads to a loss of protein. In addition, encourage the patient to take a balanced diet with a good supply of calories, vitamins and minerals to support the healing process. A dietician will advise on the best diet for individual needs including whether supplements are required.

> We proteins really deliver when patients with non-healing wounds lose too much of us due to excessive exudate.

. . . And eat your veggies

Vegetable protein powder sprinkled into food and drinks can increase the protein content in the patient's diet without affecting the taste of the food. Protein shakes and bars are also good options for increasing protein in the diet.

He's got no taste

Keep in mind that chemotherapy and radiation can alter a patient's sense of taste. For example, some chemotherapeutic drugs will cause a metallic taste in the mouth. The GI disturbances commonly caused by chemotherapy and radiation, such as nausea, vomiting and ulcerations, can lower a patient's tolerance for foods. In addition, the psychological effects of a life-threatening illness coupled with a non-healing wound can cause anorexia and malnourishment.

Patient education

Focus on symptom management when educating a patient with a non-healing wound. Instruct the patient and his carers about the correct procedure for dressing changes. Because pain management is an important issue affecting the patient's quality of life, you should instruct him in how to manage his pain effectively, including premedication before dressing changes. You should also include proper nutrition and odour control in the teaching plan.

> When educating the patient with a non-healing wound, focus on symptom management.

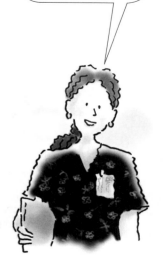

Strive for success

The success of any teaching plan relies heavily on the patient and his carers. Therefore, make sure the patient understands the plan and that it addresses any specific issues he may have. Remember that you'll need to periodically evaluate the effectiveness of your teaching plan and revise it based on your findings.

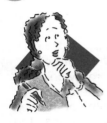

Quick quiz

1. You would suspect an infection in a non-healing wound if:
   A.   the wound bed is pink and granulation tissue is present
   B.   epithelial migration across the wound bed is delayed
   C.   small-to-moderate amounts of serous drainage are present
   D.   non-viable tissue is absent.

Answer: B. Epithelial migration is important in the normal wound healing process. A delay in epithelial migration indicates a potential infection.

2. Hypergranulation has been linked to what?
   A.   high oxygen levels in the wound bed
   B.   non-viable tissue in the wound bed
   C.   chronic inflammation, wound hypoxia and high bacterial burden
   D.   excess exudate.

Answer: C. The exact cause is not known but hypergranulation has been linked to chronic inflammation, wound hypoxia and high bacterial burden.

3. The T.I.M.E. acronym stands for:
   A.   temperature, inflammation, management and edge
   B.   tissue, infection, management and exudate
   C.   tissue, iatrogenic, moisture and exudate
   D.   tissue, inflammation/infection, moisture and edge.

Answer: D. The T.I.M.E. acronym stands for tissue, inflammation/infection, moisture and edge.

4. You can prevent bleeding in a wound by:
   A.   applying wound gels
   B.   using non-adherent dressings
   C.   applying topical anaesthetics
   D.   using hydrocolloid dressings.

Answer: B. Non-adherent dressings reduce trauma to the wound bed and reduce bleeding.

5. A nurse is providing education to a group of patients with cancer about management of their non-healing wounds. It's important for the nurse to:
   A.   review the patients' treatment plans
   B.   consider individual wound management priorities
   C.   verify the types of cancer
   D.   determine the locations of the wounds.

Answer: B. The nurse must consider what issues are important to each patient in order to improve concordance.

6. A patient informs the nurse that they lost their job because of excessive absences related to their wound. The nurse would:
   A. evaluate the patient's understanding of their wound management
   B. explain to the patient that they can no longer be seen at the clinic without a job
   C. encourage the patient to express their feelings about the job loss
   D. contact social services to assist the patient with accessing available resources.

Answer: C and D. Job loss and subsequent loss of income can be an important factor in non-concordance with wound management, which can lead to delayed wound healing. Understanding how the patient feels about this is an important step in helping them manage the issues.

Scoring

☆☆☆ If you answered all six questions correctly, give yourself a pat on the back! You've mastered the basics of non-healing wounds.

☆☆ If you answered five questions correctly, it's a 'non' issue! You're doing just fine.

☆ If you answered fewer than five questions correctly, you aren't at risk! A quick review will heal your score in no time.

References

Briggs, M. and Nelson, E.A. (2001) *Topical Agents or Dressings for Pain in Venous Leg Ulcers*. Oxford: The Cochrane Library, Issue 1.

Dowsett, C. (2008) Using the TIME framework in wound bed preparation. *British Journal of Community Nursing. Wound Care Suppl* 13(6):S15–S22.

Haisfield-Wolfe, M.E. and Rund, C. (1997) Malignant cutaneous wounds – a management protocol. *Ostomy Wound Management* 43(1):56–58, 60, 62.

Paul, J.C. and Pieper, B.A.(2008) Topical metronidazole for the treatment of wound odor: a review of the iterature. *Ostomy Wound Management* 54(3):18–27.

Segal, H.C., Hunt, B.J. and Gilding, K. (1998) The effects of alginate and non-alginate wound dressings on blood coagulation and platelet activation. *Journal of Biomaterials Applications* 12(3):249–257.

Senecal, S.J. (1999) Pain management of wound care. *Nursing Clinics of North America* 34(4):847–860.

World Health Organization (2008) *Pain Relief Ladder*. [on-line] [Accessed 6 August 2008]. Available: http://www.who.int/cancer/palliative/painladder/en/

World Union of Wound Healing Societies (2004) *Principles of Best Practice – Minimising Pain at Wound Dressing Related Procedures. A Consensus Document*. London: MEP. Available: http://www.wuwhs.org/general_publications.php

Just the facts

In this chapter, you'll learn:

♦ causes of pressure ulcers

♦ factors that increase pressure ulcer risk and ways to identify them

♦ ways to prevent pressure ulcers

♦ pressure ulcer assessment and staging criteria

♦ treatment options.

A look at pressure ulcers

Pressure ulcers are a serious health problem. Although prevalence figures vary widely because of differences in methodology, setting and subjects, approximately 18–20% of the hospitalised population suffer from chronic pressure ulcers (EPUAP 2002). Although this finding is significant in itself, prevalence in some groups – such as patients with spinal cord injuries, patients in intensive care units and nursing home residents – is much higher.

At what cost?

Although prevalence statistics vary, what has become evident are the costs associated with pressure ulcers – the cost to patients in terms of suffering and diminished quality of life, the cost to the NHS in terms of resources consumed and manpower hours to manage the problem, and the monetary cost to individuals, health insurers and government agencies. Posnett and Franks (2007) suggest that the total cost of pressure ulcers in the UK at 2005/2006 prices is between £1760 million and £2640 million.

As pressure ulcers are a chronic condition that are hard to heal and tend to recur frequently, prevention and early intervention are critical for more effective management.

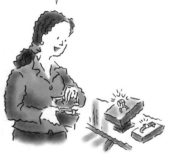

How much does this cost?! More important than money, pressure ulcers cost patients their quality of life.

The closer you get

Better disease management in pressure ulcer cases depends on closer collaboration among healthcare professionals, patients and their families/carers. All those involved are paying closer attention to prevention and the effectiveness of interventions, and they're finding better methods of quantifying and disseminating results. Pressure ulcers of category II and above are now a reportable critical incident according to NICE guidelines (NICE 2005).

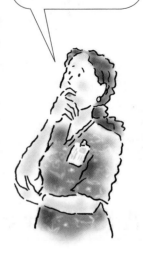

Closed pressure ulcers are unique and potentially life-threatening. Prompt recognition is difficult yet crucial.

Causes

Pressure ulcers are caused primarily by three external mechanical forces: pressure, shear and friction. They are chronic wounds (wounds that are a result of underlying pathology, fail to heal in a timely manner, resist treatment and tend to reoccur) resulting from necrosis (tissue death) due to prolonged, irreversible ischaemia brought on by compression of soft tissue. Technically speaking, pressure ulcers are the clinical manifestation of localised necrosis due to a lack of blood flow in areas under pressure.

Shades of tolerance

Different tissues have different tolerances for compression. Muscle and fat have comparatively low tolerances for pressure, whereas skin has a somewhat higher tolerance. All cells, regardless of tissue type, depend on blood circulation for the oxygen and nutrients they need. Tissue compression interferes with circulation, reducing or completely cutting off blood flow. The result, known as ischaemia, is that cells fail to receive adequate supplies of oxygen and nutrients. Unless the pressure is relieved, cells eventually die. By the time inflammation signals impending necrosis on the surface of the skin, it's likely that necrosis has occurred in deeper tissues.

Location, location, location

Pressure ulcers are most common in areas where pressure compresses soft tissue over a bony prominence. (See *Areas at risk of pressure damage*, page 163.) The tissue is pinched between the outer pressure and the hard underlying surface. Other factors that contribute to the problem include shear, friction and, to some extent, moisture, which increases the susceptibility of the skin to trauma. Planning effective interventions for prevention and treatment requires a sound understanding of pressure ulcer causes.

Areas at risk of pressure damage

The illustration below shows the areas most at risk of pressure damage.

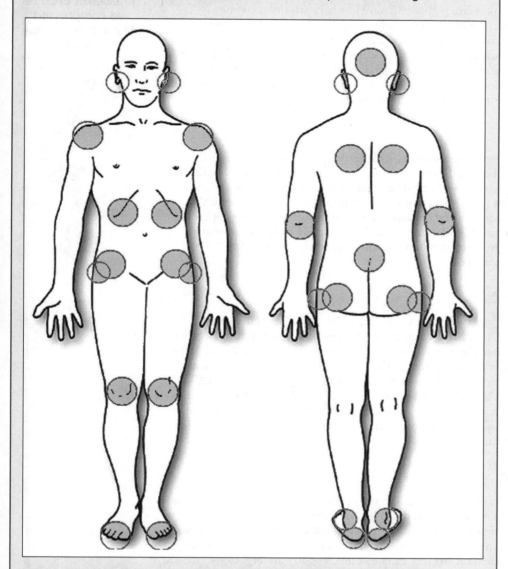

Reproduced with permission of the European Pressure Ulcer Advisory Panel (EPUAP) 2009.

Pressure

Capillaries are connected to arteries and veins through intermediary vessels called arterioles and venules. In healthy individuals, capillary filling pressure is about 32 mmHg where arterioles connect to capillaries and 12 mmHg where capillaries connect to venules. Therefore, external pressure greater than capillary filling pressure can cause problems. In frail or ill people, capillary filling pressures may be much lower. External pressure that exceeds capillary perfusion pressure compresses blood vessels and causes ischaemia in the tissues supplied by those vessels.

When external pressure exceeds capillary filling pressure, I become so compressed that ischaemia may result.

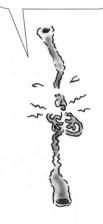

Tip of the iceberg

If the pressure continues long enough, capillaries collapse and thrombose and toxic metabolic by-products accumulate. Cells in nearby muscle and subcutaneous tissues begin to die. Muscle and fat are less tolerant of interruptions in blood flow than skin. Consequently, by the time signs of impending necrosis appear on the skin, underlying tissue has probably suffered substantial damage. Keep this in mind when assessing the size of a pressure ulcer.

The pressure mounts

When external pressure exceeds venous capillary refill pressure (about 12 mmHg), capillaries begin to leak. The resulting oedema increases the amount of pressure on blood vessels, further impeding circulation. When interstitial pressure surpasses arterial pressure, blood is forced into nearby tissues which appear warm and red (non-blanchable erythema). Continued capillary occlusion, lack of oxygen and nutrients and build-up of toxic waste leads to necrosis of muscle, subcutaneous tissue and, ultimately, the dermis and epidermis.

Spreading the load

The simplest way to reduce the pressure is to distribute it across as large a surface area as possible. For example, the force exerted on the buttocks of a person lying in bed is about 70 mmHg. However, when the same person sits on a hard surface, the force exerted on the ischial tuberosities can be as much as 300 mmHg. Consequently, bony prominences are particularly susceptible to pressure ulcers; however, they aren't the only areas at risk. Ulcers can develop on any soft tissue subjected to prolonged pressure.

Understanding the pressure gradient

In this illustration, the V-shaped pressure gradient results from the upwards force exerted by the supporting surface and the downwards force of the bony prominence. Pressure is greatest on tissues at the apex of the gradient and lessens to the right and left of this point.

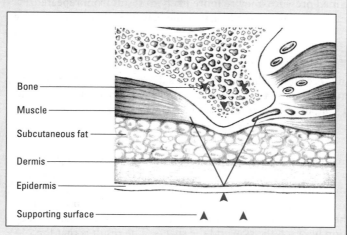

Bone
Muscle
Subcutaneous fat
Dermis
Epidermis
Supporting surface

Between a bone and a hard place

When blood vessels, muscle, subcutaneous fat and skin are compressed between a bone and an external surface – a bed or chair, for instance – pressure is exerted on the tissues from both the external surface and the bone. In effect, the external surface produces pressure and the bone produces counter pressure. These opposing forces create a cone-shaped pressure gradient. (See *Understanding the pressure gradient.*) Although the pressure affects all tissues between these two points, tissues closest to the bony prominence suffer the greatest damage.

Under pressure

Over time, pressure and the resulting hypoxia causes a growing discomfort that prompts a person to change position before tissue ischaemia occurs. In ulcer formation, an inverse relationship exists between time and pressure. Typically, low pressure for long periods is far more damaging than high pressure for short periods. For example, a pressure of 70 mmHg sustained for 2 hours or longer almost always causes irreversible tissue damage, whereas a pressure of 240 mmHg can be endured for a short time with little or no tissue damage. Furthermore, after the time–pressure

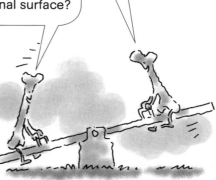

Did you know that we bones produce counter-pressure when pressure is exerted on tissues from an external surface?

I don't know anything about that but I do know that if you don't exert some pressure right now, I'll be stuck up here all day!

threshold for damage passes, damage continues even after the pressure stops. Although pressure ulcers can result from one period of sustained pressure, they're more likely to result from repeated ischaemic events without adequate time between events for recovery.

Shear

Shearing force intensifies the pressure's destructive effects. Shear is a mechanical force that runs parallel, rather than perpendicular, to an area of skin; deep tissues feel the brunt of the force.

The shear truth

Shearing force is most likely to develop during repositioning or when a patient slides down after being placed in a semi recumbent position. However, simply elevating the head of the bed increases shear and pressure in the sacral and coccygeal areas because gravity pulls the body down but the skin on the back resists the motion due to friction between the skin and the sheets. The result is that the skeleton (and attached tissues) actually slides somewhat beneath the skin (evidenced by the puckering of skin in the gluteal area), generating shearing force between outer layers of tissue and deeper layers. The force generated is enough to obstruct, tear, stretch and narrow blood vessels. (See *Shearing force*, page 167.)

As a result of this narrowing of the vessels, shearing force reduces the length of time that tissue can endure a given pressure before ischaemia or necrosis occurs. A sufficiently high level of shearing force can halve the amount of pressure needed to produce vascular occlusion. Research indicates that shearing force is responsible for the high incidence of triangular-shaped sacral ulcers and the large areas of tunneling or deep undermining beneath these ulcers.

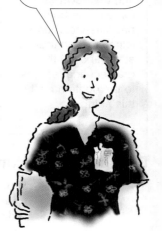

Be aware that a sufficiently high level of shearing force can have the amount of pressure needed to produce vascular occlusion.

Friction

Friction is another potentially damaging mechanical force. Friction develops as one surface moves across another surface – for example, the patient's skin sliding across the bed sheet. Abrasions are wounds created by friction.

Friction prediction

Those at particularly high risk for tissue damage due to friction include patients who have uncontrollable movements or spastic conditions, patients who wear braces or appliances that rub against the skin and older patients. Friction is also a problem for patients who have trouble lifting themselves during repositioning. Rubbing

Shearing force

Shear is a mechanical force parallel, rather than perpendicular, to an area of tissue. In this illustration, gravity pulls the body down the incline of the bed. The skeleton and attached tissues move, but the skin remains stationary, held in place by friction between the skin and the bed linen. The skeleton and attached tissues actually slide within the skin, causing skin to pucker in the gluteal area.

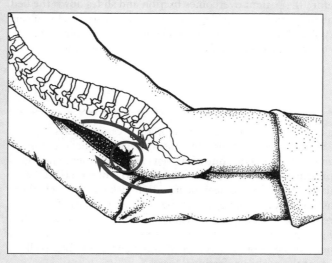

against the sheet can result in an abrasion, which increases the potential for deeper tissue damage. Elevating the head of the bed, as discussed earlier, generates friction between the patient's skin and the bed linen as gravity tugs the patient's body downwards. As the skeleton moves inside the skin, friction and shearing force combine to increase the risk of tissue damage in the sacral area. Dry lubricants such as skin protectants and adherent dressings with slippery backings can help reduce the impact of friction. The use of talcum powder on the skin should be avoided but it may be suitable to put on the surface of devices such as dressings and splints. Perhaps the most important aspect of reducing the impact of friction is the use of appropriate moving and handling equipment such as glide sheets and hoists.

Moisture

Prolonged exposure to moisture can waterlog or macerate skin. Maceration contributes to pressure ulcer formation by softening the connective tissue. Macerated epidermis erodes more easily, particularly when subjected to friction, degenerates and, eventually,

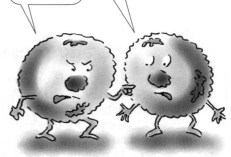

sloughs off. In addition, damp skin adheres to bed linen more readily, making the effects of shear more profound as it increase the time before the patient overcomes friction and slides down the bed. Consequently, moist skin is five times more likely to develop ulcers than dry skin. Excessive moisture can result from perspiration, wound drainage, bathing or faecal or urinary incontinence.

Risk factors

Factors that increase the risk of developing pressure ulcers include advancing age, immobility, incontinence, infection, non-blanching erythema, poor nutrition, sensory impairment and low blood pressure. Patients with peripheral arterial disease (PAD) are particularly susceptible to heel ulcers. High-risk patients, whether in an institution or at home, should be assessed regularly for pressure ulcers. Assessing an individual's risk should involve both clinical judgement and structured assessment procedures. All formal assessment of risk should be recorded and made accessible to all members of the multi-professional team.

Age

The risk of developing pressure ulcers increases with age because ageing affects all aspects of healing. (See *Age and pressure ulcers*.)

Immobility

Immobility may be the greatest risk factor for pressure ulcer development. The patient's ability to move in response to pressure sensations as well as the frequency with which their position is

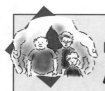

Handle with care

Age and pressure ulcers

With advancing age, the skin becomes more fragile as epidermal turnover slows, vascularisation decreases and skin layers adhere less securely to one another. Older adults have less lean body mass and less subcutaneous tissue cushioning bony areas. Consequently, they're more likely to suffer tissue damage due to friction, shear and pressure. Other common problems that can contribute to pressure ulcer development in elderly patients include poor nutrition, poor hydration and impaired respiratory or immune systems.

changed should always be considered in risk assessment. Patients with a body mass index (BMI) of greater than 30 are especially at risk because of their additional weight and reduced independence, they are also at risk because of the difficulties experienced when moving and handling them.

Incontinence

Incontinence increases a patient's exposure to moisture and, over time, increases the risk of skin breakdown. Both urinary and faecal incontinence create problems as a result of excessive moisture and chemical irritation. Due to pathogens in the stool, faecal incontinence can cause more skin damage than urinary incontinence. The chemical interaction between urine and faeces results in a greatly increased risk of damage in those who are doubly incontinent.

Moisture lesions

Recently, emphasis has been clearly placed on differentiating between ulceration caused by pressure and wounds caused by moisture, particularly incontinence. This is an important distinction as although moisture contributes to the risk of pressure ulcer formation, management of moisture lesions is very different to the management of pressure ulcers. (See *Pressure ulcer or moisture lesion?*)

Pressure ulcer or moisture lesion?

	Pressure ulcer	Moisture lesion
Causes	Evidence/history of pressure, shear or friction	Skin obviously moist, history of incontinence
Position	Usually over a bony prominence unless compressed with equipment such as a catheter or oxygen mask	Not over bone, frequently in the natal cleft and/or over the buttocks. May present as 'kissing' or copy lesion with the shape/pattern on both buttocks
Shape	Usually distinct shape with obvious edges, 1 or 2 wounds	Frequently multiple wounds with diffuse edges
Depth	From superficial to deep, may be down to bone	Usually superficial – unless it becomes infected
Necrosis	Frequently necrotic tissue present as hypoxia causes necrosis	No necrosis, damage is caused by overhydration which does not result in necrosis
Edges	Distinct edges, may be rolled or raised in chronic stages	Edges may be difficult to determine, jagged edges are seen in moisture lesions that have been subjected to friction

(EPUAP 2005)

Non-blanching erythema (NBE)

Patients who have non-blanching erythema are considered to be at high risk of further pressure damage and the presence of NBE has been found to be both a warning signal and as accurate a predictor of future damage as a recognised risk assessment tool.

Nutrition

Proper nutrition is vitally important to tissue integrity. A strong correlation exists between poor nutrition and pressure ulceration. Don't overlook the importance of nutrition during treatment. (See Chapter 1, *Nutrition*, page 19.)

Albumin acumen

Increased protein is required for the body to heal itself. Albumin is one of the key proteins in the body. A patient's serum albumin level is an important indicator of their protein levels. A subnormal serum albumin level is a late manifestation of protein deficiency. Normal serum albumin levels range from 3.5 to 5 g/dl. Serum albumin deficits are ranked as follows:

- mild – 3 to 3.5 g/dl
- moderate – 2.5 to 3 g/dl
- severe – less than 2.5 g/dl.

Handle with care

Pressure ulcers in patients with a high BMI

Patients with a high BMI (>30) are at risk for pressure ulcer development for several reasons:

- They're nutritional status may not be optimal.
- They're prone to developing protein malnutrition during metabolic stress (even though they may have excess body fat storage).
- They often have decreased vascularity in adipose tissue.
- They're unable to change position or move independently due to immobility.
- The moist environment in skin folds promotes bacterial growth, which can lead to fungal infections. This decreased skin integrity also predisposes patients to pressure ulcer development.

The EPUAP nutritional guidelines (EPUAP 2003) state that the primary goal of nutritional intervention is to correct protein–energy malnutrition. General guidance would be that an individual would require a minimum of 30–35 kcal per kg body weight per day, with 1–1.5 g/kg/day of protein required and 1 ml per cal of fluid intake. When aiming to correct nutritional deficiency, oral feeding should always be the first option followed by oral supplementation and then tube feeding. Whilst there is good evidence to support the role of protein replenishment/supplementation, the value of vitamins and trace element supplementation is less clear.

PAD

Peripheral arterial disease causes a reduced blood supply to the extremities, where tissues are poorly perfused they are much more susceptible to hypoxia and ultimately tissue death. Heels have a poor protective covering with there being little tissue between the bone and the skin, therefore when the tissues are also poorly perfused this becomes a very vulnerable area.

Sensory impairment

Patients who have reduced or loss of sensation will not receive the signal to move in response to pressure. They may not be aware of the presence of hard items (e.g. catheters, splints, oxygen tubing or masks and too tight bandages/stockings) which will cause damage to the skin.

Blood pressure

Low arterial blood pressure is clearly linked to tissue ischaemia, particularly in patients with vascular disease. When blood pressure is low, the body shunts blood away from the peripheral vascular system that serves the skin and towards vital organs to ensure their health. As perfusion drops, the skin is less tolerant of sustained external pressure and the risk of damage due to ischaemia rises. Equally, a patient who is hypotensive will have a lower capillary closing pressure as there is less pressure being exerted by the heart to keep the vessel open – therefore less external pressure is required to occlude it.

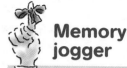

Memory jogger

To remember the five factors commonly used to determine a patient's risk of developing pressure ulcers, think of the five **I's**:

Immobility

Inactivity

Incontinence

Improper nutrition (malnutrition)

Impaired mental status or sensation.

Risk factor assessment

Several assessment tools are available to help determine a patient's risk of pressure ulcers, including the Waterlow Pressure Ulcer Risk Assessment Scale (Waterlow 2005) – the most widely used pressure ulcer assessment tool in the UK – and the Braden scale

Waterlow pressure ulcer prevention treatment policy

RING SCORES IN TABLE, ADD TOTAL. MORE THAN 1 SCORE/CATEGORY CAN BE USED

BUILD/WEIGHT FOR HEIGHT	◆	SKIN TYPE VISUAL RISK AREAS	◆	SEX AGE	◆	MALNUTRITION SCREENING TOOL (MST) (Nutrition Vol.15, No.6 1999–Australia	
AVERAGE BMI = 20–24.9	0	HEALTHY	0	MALE	1	A– HAS PATIENT LOST WEIGHT RECENTLY	B–WEIGHT LOSS SCORE
		TISSUE PAPER	1	FEMALE	2		0.5–5 kg = 1
ABOVE AVERAGE BMI = 25–29.9	1	DRY	1	14–49	1	YES – GO TO B	5–10 kg = 2
		OEDEMATOUS	1	50–64	2	NO – GO TO C	10–15 kg = 3
OBESE BMI > 30	2	CLAMMY, PYREXIA	1	65–74	3	UNSURE – GO TO C AND	>15 kg = 4
BELOW AVERAGE BMI < 20	3	DISCOLOURED GRADE 1	2	75–80	4	SCORE 2	UNSURE = 2
BMI = Wt (Kg)/Ht (m)^2				81+	5	C–PATIENT EATING POORLY OR LACK OF APPETITE 'NO' = 0; 'YES' SCORE = 1	NUTRITION SCORE If > 2 refer for nutrition assessment / intervention
		BROKEN/SPOTS GRADE 2–4	3				

CONTINENCE	◆	MOBILITY	◆	SPECIAL RISKS				
COMPLETE/ CATHETERIZED	0	FULLY	0	TISSUE MALNUTRITION	◆	NEUROLOGICAL DEFICIT		◆
URINE INCONTINENCE	1	RESTLESS/FIDGETY	1	TERMINAL CACHEXIA	8	DIABETES, MULTIPLE SCHLEROSIS, CEREBROVASCULAR ACCIDENT		4–6
FAECAL INCONTINENCE	2	APATHETIC	2	MULTIPLE ORGAN FAILURE	8			
		RESTRICTED	3	SINGLE ORGAN FAILURE (RESPIRATORY RENAL, CARDIAC)	5	MOTOR/SENSORY		4–6
URINARY + FAECAL INCONTINENCE	3	BEDBOUND e.g. TRACTION	4			PARAPLEGIA (MAX OF 6)		4–6
		CHAIRBOUND e.g. WHEELCHAIR	5	PERIPHERAL VASCULAR DISEASE	5	MAJOR SURGERY or TRAUMA		
SCORE						ORTHOPAEDIC/SPINAL		5
10+ AT RISK				ANAEMIA (Hb < 8)	2	ON TABLE > 2 HR#		5
15+ HIGH RISK				SMOKING	1	ON TABLE > 6 HR#		8
20+ VERY HIGH RISK				MEDICATION—CYTOTOXICS, LONG-TERM/HIGH-DOSE STEROIDS, ANTI-INFLAMMATORY MAX OF 4				

\# Scores can be discounted after 48 hours provided patient is recovering normally

© J Waterlow 1985 Revised 2005*

Obtainable from the Nook, Stoke Road, Henlade TAUNTON TA3 5LX

* The 2005 revision incorporates the research undertaken by Queensland Health.   www. judy-waterlow.co.uk

REMEMBER TISSUE DAMAGE MAY START PRIOR TO ADMISSION IN CASUALTY. A SEATED PATIENT IS AT RISK ASSESSMENT IF THE PATIENT FALLS INTO ANY OF THE RISK CATEGORIES, THEN PREVENTATIVE NURSING IS REQUIRED. A COMBINATION OF GOOD NURSING TECHNIQUES AND PREVENTATIVE AIDS WILL BE NECESSARY

ALL ACTIONS MUST BE DOCUMENTED

PREVENTION

PRESSURE REDUCING AIDS

Special Mattress/beds: 10+ Overlays or specialist foam mattresses.

15+ Alternating pressure overlays, mattresses and bed systems

20+ Bed systems: Fluidized bead, low air loss and alternating pressure mattresses

Note: Preventative aids cover a wide spectrum of specialist features. Efficacy should be judged, if possible, on the basis of independent evidence.

Cushions: No person should sit in a wheelchair without some form of cushioning. If nothing else is available—use the person's own pillow. (Consider infection risk)

10+ 100 mm foam cushion

15+ Specialist gel and/or foam cushion

20+ Specialized cushion, adjustable to individual person.

Bed clothing: Avoid plastic draw sheets, inco pads and tightly tucked in sheet/sheet covers, especially when using specialist bed and mattress overlay systems

Use duvet – plus vapour-permeable membrane.

NURSING CARE

General Hand washing, frequent changes of position, lying, sitting. Use of pillows

Pain Appropriate pain control

Nutrition High protein, vitamins and minerals

Patient Handling Correct lifting technique – hoists – monkey poles. Transfer devices

Patient Comfort Aids Real Sheepskin – bed cradle

Operating Table

Theatre/A&E Trolley 100 mm (4 ins) cover plus adequate protection

Skin Care General hygene, NO rubbing, cover with an appropriate dressing

WOUND GUIDELINES

Assessment Odour, exudate, measure/photograph position

WOUND CLASSIFICATION - EPUAP

GRADE 1 Discoloration of intact skin not affected by light finger pressure (non-blanching erythema)

This may be difficult to identify in darkly-pigmented skin

GRADE 2 Partial-thickness skin loss or damage involving epidermis and/or dermis

The pressure ulcer is superficial and presents clinically as an abrasion, blister or shallow crater

GRADE 3 Full-thickness skin loss involving damage of subcutaneous tissue but not extending to the underlying fascia

The pressure ulcer presents clinically as a deep crater with or without undermining of adjacent tissue

GRADE 4 Full-thickness skin loss with extensive destruction and necrosis extending to underlying tissue.

Dressing Guide Use local dressings formulary and/or www.worldwidewounds

IF TREATMENT IS REQUIRED, FIRST REMOVE PRESSURE

(Bergstrom *et al.* 1998). (See *Waterlow pressure ulcer prevention treatment policy*, page 172.) The Waterlow scale scores a range of factors including: Build/weight for height (BMI), continence staus, skin type/ visible risk areas, sex, age, malnutrition screening (using the MST tool) and special risk categories such as tissue malnutrition, neurological deficit and surgery/trauma. Additional risk can be noted for patients on particular medications such as long-term steroids or sedatives. With the Waterlow score, a higher number denotes a higher level of risk. The Braden scale scores aetiological factors that contribute to prolonged pressure as well as factors that contribute to diminished tissue tolerance for pressure, including sensory perception, moisture, activity, mobility, nutrition, friction and shear. With the Braden, a lower score denotes a higher level of risk.

Common denominators

Most scales use the following factors to determine a patient's risk of developing pressure ulcers:
- immobility
- inactivity
- incontinence
- malnutrition
- impaired mental status or sensation.

Each category receives a value based on the patient's condition. The sum of these values determines the patient's score and level of risk. Scores for each category as well as the assessment as a whole help the healthcare team develop appropriate interventions. Most healthcare facilities require an assessment score for every patient admitted. NICE guidance (NICE 2005) recommends using a validated tool, the most frequently used in the UK and Europe are the Waterlow scale and the Braden Scale.

Early bird

In nursing home populations, most pressure ulcers develop during the 2 weeks immediately following admission, so early identification of at-risk patients is crucial. No definitive guidelines exist for how often to reassess a patient; however, use a common-sense approach, such as reassessing the patient when their condition changes or in the event that they becomes chair-bound or bedridden.

Prevention

Pressure ulcer prevention focuses on compensating for prevailing risk factors and addressing the underlying pathophysiology, including managing pressure, skin integrity and nutrition. When planning interventions, be sure to adopt a holistic approach and consider all of the patient's needs.

Managing pressure

Managing the intensity and duration of pressure is a fundamental goal in prevention, especially for patients with mobility limitations. Frequent, careful repositioning helps the patient avoid the damaging repetitive pressure that can cause tissue ischaemia and subsequent necrosis. When repositioning the patient, it's important to reduce the duration and intensity of pressure.

Positioning

Any time the patient is repositioned, the skin and particularly vulnerable areas such as the heels, elbows and sacrum should be checked for areas of reddened skin. Avoid the use of doughnut-shaped supports or ring cushions that encircle the ischaemic area because these can reduce blood flow to an even wider expanse of tissue. If the affected area is on an extremity, use appropriate support systems to elevate the limb and reduce pressure. Avoid raising the head of the bed more than 30 degrees to prevent tissue damage due to friction and shearing force.

Your patient may not be quite ready to do the limbo yet but, remember, inactivity increases their risk of pressure ulcer development.

Baby steps

Inactivity increases a patient's risk of ulcer development. To the degree that the patient is physically able, encourage activity. Start with a short step – help them out of bed and into a chair. As tolerance improves, help them walk around the room and then a little further. Remember, patients can be quite active without actually getting out of bed, some change in position is better than none. If they have an electric bed frame, a substantial position change can be achieved by raising or lowering the bed head and/or the leg section.

Positioning a patient in bed

When the patient is on their side, avoid positioning them directly on the greater trochanter of the femur. Instead, tilt the patient through 30 degrees and put the weight onto the buttock, use pillows or a foam wedge to maintain the position, ensure that the patient is comfortable and well supported and not left in a twisted position. This position ensures that no pressure is placed on the trochanter or sacrum. Also, place a pillow between the knees and ankles to minimise the pressure exerted when one limb lies on top of the other. (See *Repositioning a reclining patient*, page 176.)

Repositioning a reclining patient

When repositioning a reclining patient, use the Rule of 30, raising the head of the bed 30 degrees (as shown). Avoid raising the head of the bed more than 30 degrees to prevent buildup of shearing pressure. When you must raise it more – at meal times, for instance – keep the periods brief.

As you reposition the patient from their left side to their right side, make sure the weight rests on the buttock, not the hip bone. This reduces pressure on the trochanter and sacrum. The angle between the bed and an imaginary lateral line through their hips should be about 30 degrees. If needed, use pillows or a foam wedge to help the patient maintain the proper position (as shown). Cushion pressure points, such as the knees or shoulders, with pillows.

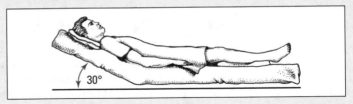

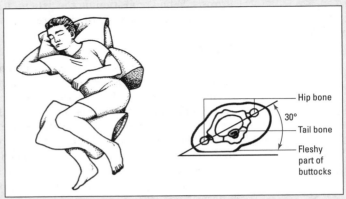

Suspending the heel is ideal

Heels present a particularly difficult challenge. Even with the aid of specially designed mattresses, reducing the pressure on heels to below capillary refill pressure is almost impossible. Instead, suspend the patient's foot so that the bony prominence on the heel is under no pressure. A foam or air-filled boot may be used in bed or chair although this may limit mobility. Polymer gel heel pads (e.g. Dermal Pads™) may also help redistribute pressure, and as they are smaller and less cumbersome may be more comfortable for the patient. Remember to take care to avoid knee contraction if elevating the heels – there is often a natural tendency to also bend the knees, therefore, the legs should be supported along the full length to prevent this occurring.

Positioning a seated patient

A patient is more likely to develop pressure ulcers from sitting than from being in bed. Sitting tends to focus all of the patient's weight on the relatively small surface areas of the buttocks, thighs and soles of the feet. Much of this weight is focused on the small area of tissue covering the ischial tuberosities. Proper posture and alignment help ensure that the weight of the patient's body is distributed as evenly as possible.

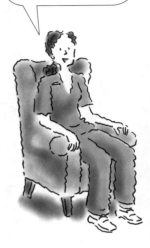

Proper posture when sitting is a key part of pressure ulcer prevetion.

Proper posture preferred

Proper posture alone can significantly reduce the patient's risk of ulcers. To encourage a good posture, the chair must be the correct size, the height from seat to floor should allow the patient to have their feet squarely on the floor; a seat height that is too low tips the weight back onto the coccyx and a seat height that is too high will result in the patient sliding forwards to put their feet securely on the floor. The length (or depth) of the seat is also important, a short seat will result in high pressures on the backs of the legs, a seat that is too long will again result in the patient shuffling forwards, to sit comfortably and result in an insecure position.

Be sure to include these points when explaining proper posture to the patient:
• Sit with your back erect and against the back of the chair, thighs parallel to the floor, knees comfortably parted and arms horizontal and supported by the arms of the chair. (This posture distributes weight evenly over the available body surface area.)
• Keep your feet flat on the floor to protect your heels from focused pressure and distribute the weight of your legs over the largest available surface area – the soles.
• Avoid slouching, which causes shearing force and friction and places undue pressure on the sacrum and coccyx.
• Keep your thighs and arms parallel to ensure that weight is evenly distributed all along your thighs and forearms instead of being focused on the ischial tuberosities and elbows, respectively.
• Part your knees to keep knees and ankles from rubbing together.

Put your feet up

If the patient likes to use a footstool, check to see if their knees are positioned above the level of their hips. If so, it means that the weight has shifted from the back of their thighs to the ischial tuberosities. This is the same problem that occurs if the chair itself is too short for the patient. In this case, recommend the use of a different footstool or chair. Ensure that the length of the leg is supported rather than simply resting the heels on the stool which can increase the risk of heel ulcers.

Turn the other cheek

Patients at risk should reposition themselves every 15 minutes while sitting, if they can. Patients with spinal cord injuries can perform wheelchair push-ups to intermittently relieve pressure on the buttocks and sacrum; however, this requires a fair amount of upper body strength. Others may have injuries that preclude

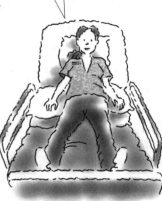

A pillow is good for support but it isn't your only option.

using this technique. Repositioning in the chair can be as simple as leaning forwards onto a table for a short time so that the weight is lifted from the coccyx, if they are able, the patient can also lean to each side for a short time to relieve pressure from each ischial tuberosity.

Support aids and cushions

There are a vast array of support surfaces and cushioning pads. Special beds, mattresses and seating options that employ foams, gels, water and air as cushioning agents make it possible to tailor a comprehensive and personal system of supports for the patient. Remember, equipment provision should cover the whole 24 hour period and not simply when the patient is in bed. Effective care depends on knowledge of the classes and types of products available. (See *Pressure redistribution devices*.)

Pressure redistribution devices

Here are some special mattresses and beds that help reduce or redistribute pressure when a patient is confined to one position for long periods.

Air-fluidised beds

Beads move under an airflow to support the patient, thus reducing shearing force and friction.

Alternating-pressure air mattress

Alternating deflation and inflation of mattress tubes changes areas of pressure.

Electronic bed frames

Electronic bed frames can help patients move their own position and can be used to prevent shearing and friction forces.

Foot cradle

A foot cradle lifts the bed linen to relieve pressure over the feet.

Gel pads

Gel pads disperse pressure over a wide surface area and are mainly used in theatres.

Low-air-loss beds

Inflated air cushions adjust for optimal pressure relief for the patient's body size.

Moving and handling devices

Lift sheets and other mechanical lifting devices prevent shearing by lifting the patient rather than dragging them across the bed.

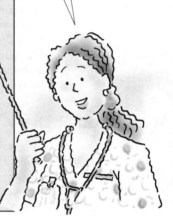

The more you learn about available options, the better prepared you are to best care for your patient.

False security

Be informed, but be cautious as well. Using these devices can instil a false sense of security. It's important to remember that as helpful as these devices may be, they aren't substitutes for attentive care. Patients require individual turning schedules regardless of the equipment used, and this schedule depends on an assessment of the patient's tolerance for pressure. All the other factors which contribute to risk such as malnutrition and incontinence should also be addressed.

Horizontal support

Horizontal support surfaces include beds, mattresses and mattress overlays. These products employ foams, gels and air to minimise the pressure a patient experiences while lying in bed.

Beds

Specialty beds, such as oscillating and rotation beds, relieve pressure by rotating the patient or helping to lift the patient to reduce the risk of friction and shear. They also promote postural drainage and peristalsis. However, they're expensive and are rarely an option for a patient returning home. Electronic bed frames are increasingly used in hospital settings; these encourage a greater range of positions and can encourage patient participation/independence in repositioning.

Mattresses

Most mattresses worth considering use some form or manipulation of foam, gel or air, to cushion the patient. High specification foam replacement mattresses can provide the same benefits derived from a standard mattress with a foam overlay. Alternating pressure (AP) systems are the most commonly used pressure redistributing devices used in the UK. They alternately apply and remove pressure along the length of the mattress. AP systems are available as both mattress replacements and mattress overlays. They are suitable for use in both hospital and community settings. Some of the AP systems have inbuilt devices which automatically adjust to both the patient's weight and weight distribution so they will change the inflation pressures depending on if the patient is laid down (weight evenly distributed) or sat up (weight concentrated in smaller area). Low air-loss and air-fluidised/high air-loss mattresses are specialised support devices that pass air over the patient's skin. These mattresses promote evaporation and are especially useful when skin maceration is a problem. However, a risk of dehydration with the use of air-fluidised mattresses exists.

Bottoming out

If the patient's weight completely compresses a cushion, mattress or overlay, then the equipment is not giving the patient adequate support. To make sure the patient isn't bottoming out, hand check whenever a new piece of equipment is put into service or if you suspect it is not working properly. Do remember that the most common reason any electrical system malfunctions is user error, simple checks such as is the plug in and the socket switched on should be first line actions if any piece of electrical equipment alarms/malfunctions. To hand check, slide one hand – palm up and fingers outstretched – between the support surface (e.g. bed or chair) and the mattress/cushion. If you can feel the patient's body through the equipment, check the system for obvious faults including is any quick release CPR facility firmly in place, and if there are no obvious electrical faults replace the system with something more suitable for the patient's weight/weight distribution.

Vertical support

Products designed to help prevent pressure ulcers while sitting fall into two broad categories: products that reduce or redistribute pressure and products that ease repositioning.

A cushy situation

Ambulatory and wheelchair-dependent patients should use seat cushions to distribute weight over the largest possible surface area. Wheelchair-dependent patients require an especially rugged seat cushion that can stand up to the rigours of daily use. In many instances, a foam cushion that's 7.5 to 10 cm (3 to 4 inches) thick suffices.

Many wheelchair-seating clinics now use computers to create custom seating systems tailored to fit the physiology and needs of each patient. For patients with spinal cord injuries, the selection of wheelchair seating is based on pressure evaluation, lifestyle, postural stability, continence and cost. Custom seats and cushions are more expensive; however, in this case, the added expense is justifiable. Encourage wheelchair-dependent patients to replace seat cushions as soon as their current one begins to deteriorate.

A position on repositioning

Repositioning is just as important when the patient is sitting as when in bed. For a patient requiring assistance, various devices are available, including overhead frames, standing frames, trapezes and Zimmer frames. These devices can help the patient reposition themselves as necessary. In addition, healthcare personnel can help manoeuvre I.V. poles and other support equipment. Advice should be sought from the physiotherapy team about how to improve or maintain mobility.

Managing skin integrity

An effective skin integrity management plan includes regularly inspecting for tissue breakdown, routinely cleaning and moisturising and taking steps to protect the skin from incontinence, if applicable.

Inspecting the skin

Routinely inspect the patient's skin for pressure damage, depending on their assessed risk and ability to tolerate pressure. Ensure anti-embolic stockings are regularly removed (at least daily) and that patients who have bandages or plaster casts *in situ* that can not be removed daily are asked about any change in sensation or pain. Check for pallor and areas of redness – both signs of ischaemia. Be aware that reactive hyperaemia (redness that occurs after pressure is removed) is commonly the first external sign of ischaemia due to pressure. In non-white skin, redness may not be obvious, check carefully for changes in skin colour, temperature and texture.

Cleaning the skin

Usually, cleansing with a mild wash such as Dove™ and warm water suffices for daily skin hygiene. Advise the patient to use a soft cloth to pat, rather than rub, their skin dry and to avoid scrubbing or using harsh cleansing agents. In patients who require regular washing, a pH balanced cleanser, soap substitute such as Aqueous Cream BP or emollient such as Oilatum™ is preferable to soap which can strip the skin of the natural protective mantle.

Moisturising the skin

Skin becomes dry, flaky and less pliable when it loses moisture. Dry skin is more susceptible to infection and ulceration. There is a huge number of skin moisturising products available. Where possible choose the simplest product with the fewest number of ingredients. Avoid additives such as perfume which may increase the likelihood of sensitivities or skin reactions. Inexpensive products such as 50:50 (50% white soft paraffin and 50% liquid paraffin) are available in bulk and are very easy to use. Take care though; paraffin is inflammable so patients and carers should be advised to keep well away from any source of naked flame (including cigarettes/cigars).

When using moisturisers it is best to apply creams and ointments in the direction of hair growth as it helps prevent blocking and irritation of the hair follicles.

There are four categories of skin moisturisers: bath additives, lotions, creams and ointments. (See *Quick guide to moisturisers*, page 182.)

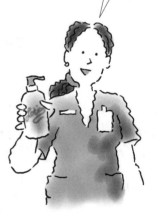

Four categories of skin moisturisers exist: bath additives, lotions, creams and ointments.

Quick guide to moisturisers

Keeping the skin moist is essential in helping to prevent pressure ulcer development, and many moisturiser products are available. Use this chart as a quick way to determine which product may be best for your patient.

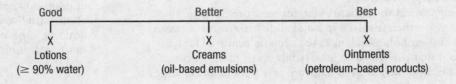

Good	Better	Best
X	X	X
Lotions	Creams	Ointments
($\geq$ 90% water)	(oil-based emulsions)	(petroleum-based products)

Bath additives

Bath additives are usually added to the bath or washing water. They prevent excessive moisture loss from the skin and are usually used in conjunction with creams and ointments. Typically, the skin is left damp before applying the cream as this traps the most moisture.

Lotions

Lotions are dissolved powder crystals held in suspension by surfactants. They have the highest water content, which is why lotions feel cool as they're applied. They also evaporate faster than any other type of moisturiser; consequently, they must be applied more often.

Creams

Creams are preparations of oil and water that are more occlusive than lotions. They don't have to be applied as often as lotions; therefore, three or four applications per day should be sufficient. Creams are better for preventing moisture loss due to evaporation than for replenishing skin moisture.

Ointments

Ointments are preparations of water in oil (typically lanolin or petroleum). They are effective for very dry skin conditions but can be greasy. They are the most occlusive and longest-lasting form of moisturiser. They take time to be absorbed and leave a visible protective barrier on the skin.

Protecting the skin

Although some moisture is good, too much can be a problem. Friction easily erodes waterlogged skin, making it more susceptible

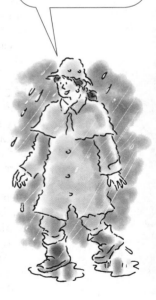

Be sure to protect your patient's skin from excessive moisture because waterlogged skin is more susceptible to bacteria.

to irritants and bacteria colonisation than dry skin. Close monitoring helps head off problems before they escalate.

Skin protection is particularly important if the patient is incontinent. Urine and faeces introduce chemical irritants and bacteria as well as moisture, which can speed skin breakdown. To effectively manage incontinence, first determine the cause and then plan interventions that protect skin integrity while addressing the underlying problem. Make use of skin barriers to protect the skin from the damaging effects of urine and faeces.

In older adults, don't assume that incontinence is a normal part of ageing. It isn't. Instead, consider factors that can precipitate incontinence, such as:
• faecal impaction and tube feeding (can cause diarrhoea)
• a reaction to medication (can cause urinary incontinence)
• urinary tract infection
• mobility problems (can keep the patient from reaching the bathroom in time)
• confusion or embarrassment (can keep the patient from asking for a bedpan or help getting to the bathroom)
• clothing barriers, such as buttons or belts can keep the patient from getting out of clothing in time.

Lend a helping hand

Whether the underlying cause is reversible, encourage the patient to ask for help when they need a bedpan or to go to the bathroom. Use incontinence collectors (bottles), removable sheaths, pants or under-pads and skin barriers as appropriate to minimise skin damage. (See *Managing incontinence*, page 184.) Step up the frequency of mobilising, toileting, inspections, cleansing and moisturising for these patients. If possible try and position the patient as close to the bathroom as possible. When using pads or pants, smoothing them prior to application helps reduce the risk of pressure damage. Care should be taken when using ointments and pads together as the ointment may coat the pad and reduce its ability to absorb.

Managing nutrition

Proper nutrition, including a balanced dietary intake and maintaining proper weight, is essential to both ulcer prevention and healing.

Dietary intake

Protein is particularly important to skin maintenance. The patient needs a balanced diet that includes about 0.8 g/kg/day of protein.

Managing incontinence

Patients experiencing incontinence require careful monitoring and special interventions to prevent skin damage caused by excessive moisture, chemical irritation or microbial infection. Three types of aid can help manage incontinence and minimise its impact on patients: incontinence collectors, incontinence pants and underpads and topical barriers.

Incontinence collectors

- Condom catheters (sheath) can help manage urinary incontinence in men (similar but less effective devices exist for women).
- Faecal incontinence collectors can be pectin skin barriers with an attached, drainable pouch (similar to colostomy pouching systems) or rectal tubes.
- Collectors need to be changed on a regular schedule and whenever a leak is detected. Faecal containment systems may be useful when patients have persistant diarrhoea (expected to last more than 3 days)

Incontinence garments and underpads

- Pants and underpads wick moisture away from the patient's skin. Underpads and pant alternatives include disposable absorbent gel pants and disposable cellulose core pants.
- Studies indicate that disposable gel pants are significantly more effective in reducing wetness and maintaining normal skin pH than other alternatives. Smoothing the surface of the pants or pads makes them more comfortable and less likely to cause pressure damage.
- Don't be tempted to put a plastic or paper linen saver under an incontinent patient; this holds moisture next to the patient's skin and compounds the problem.
- Don't secure the pad to the patient. Underpads work by absorbing wetness and allowing air to circulate over the skin, drying it.
- Pants and underpads require routine monitoring so they can be changed promptly after urination or voiding.

Topical skin barriers

- Liquid copolymer film barriers protect intact skin from the damaging effects of incontinence. They're available in aerosol form or as disposable wipes. As they dry, these products form a strong, almost plastic-like barrier on the skin's surface that isn't easily washed off during normal cleaning.

For most healthy adults, this means eating one or two 3-oz servings of protein each day in the form of meat, milk, cheese or eggs.

Body weight

Low body weight is a problem for many pressure ulcer patients. An underlying illness or anorexia can make eating undesirable or impossible. Malodour related to wound leakage can cause nausea and reduce appetite. Generally speaking, patients should be weighed weekly; however, nutritional assessment should not be based solely on weight. Oedema or excessive water retention will increase or inflate the patient's weight. If the patient's history includes an unintentional 10% weight loss in the past 3–6 months, malnutrition may be the cause. A recognised malnutrition screening tool such as MUST (Malnutrition Universal Screening Tool) should be used (Elia 2003). The BMI is more reliable than the actual weight.

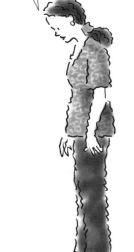

Be sure to weigh your patient weekly because low body weight is a problem for many pressure ulcer patients.

Assessment of the ulcer

Pressure ulcers can occur even with the best preventive measures. Effective treatment depends on a thorough assessment of the developing wound. Meaningful ulcer assessment requires a systematic and objective approach. First, gather the history of the ulcer, including aetiology, duration and prior treatment. (See Chapter 2, *Wound assessment and monitoring*.) The assessment should include information about the ulcer's:

- anatomical location
- characteristics (reactive hyperaemia, blanchable and non-blanchable erythema)
- size (See Chapter 2, *Dimensions*, page 42.)
- base (necrotic, sloughy, granulation or epithelial tissue)
- exudate (amount and description, is this increasing or decreasing)
- odour (this may be difficult to quantify and although it may be strong and unpleasant is not necessarily an indicator of problems, change in odour may be more significant)
- margins (sinus tracts, undermining and tunnelling)
- surrounding skin (redness, warmth, induration or hardness, swelling, signs of infection, wound edges).

Pain

Remember, in many cases, the full extent of ulceration can't be determined by visual inspection alone because there may be extensive undermining along fascial planes.

Pain drain

Before you examine the ulcer, assess the patient's pain. In most cases, pressure ulcers cause some degree of pain; in some cases, pain is severe. Have the patient rate their pain on a recognised pain assessment tool. Pain assessment should include the severity of the pain (usually on a scale of 1 to 10), the type or nature of the pain (e.g. throbbing, stabbing), the frequency of the pain (e.g. constant, procedural) and the impact of the pain on daily activities/life. (See Chapter 2, *How to assess pain*, page 36.)

Location

Ulcers are more common on the lower half of the body because it has more major bony prominences and more body weight than the upper half of the body. The most common site for pressure ulcers is the sacrum and second most frequent is the heel. However this does vary, for example, in patients who are wheelchair dependent the most common site is the ischial tuberosities and in neonates the most common site is the occiput.

Common locations for pressure ulcers include:

- sacrum
- coccyx
- ischial tuberosities
- greater trochanters
- elbows
- heels
- scapulae
- occipital bone
- sternum
- ribs
- iliac crests
- patellae
- lateral malleoli
- medial malleoli.

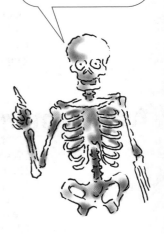

The areas over bony prominences are common pressure ulcer sites.

Characteristics categorising damage

Tissue involvement ranges from blanchable erythema to the deep destruction of tissue associated with a full-thickness wound. Pressure against tissue interrupts blood flow and causes pallor due to tissue ischaemia. If prolonged, ischaemia causes irreversible and extensive tissue damage. Following a joint review of their pressure ulcer guidelines in 2009, both the European Pressure Ulcer Advisory Panel (Europe) and the National Pressure Ulcer Advisory Panel (US) describe pressure ulcers using a 4 category classification. In addition, the US use the terms 'unclassified' and 'deep tissue injury'. Description of the extent of damage was previously referred to as staging or grading.

Reactive hyperaemia

When the pressure that causes ischaemia is released, skin flushes red as blood rushes back into the tissue. This reddening is called reactive hyperaemia. A protective mechanism in the body dilates vessels in the affected area, which increases the blood flow and speeds oxygen to starved tissues. Reactive hyperaemia first appears as a bright flush that lasts about one-half to three-quarters as long as the ischaemic period. If the applied pressure is too high for too long, reactive hyperaemia fails to meet the demand for blood, and tissue damage occurs. Usually, reactive hyperaemia is the first visible sign of ischaemia.

Blanchable erythema

Erythema (redness) results from capillary dilation near the skin's surface. In the patient with pressure ulcers, this redness results from the release of ischaemia-causing pressure. Blanchable erythema is redness that blanches (turns white) when pressed with a fingertip and then immediately turns red again when pressure is removed. This may be difficult to observe if the patient has a fast capillary refill and can be most reliably observed by pressing the area with a clean piece of see-through plastic (such as a ruler). Tissue exhibiting blanchable erythema usually resumes its normal colour within 24 hours if the pressure is removed and suffers no long-term damage; however, it can signal imminent tissue damage. The longer it takes for tissue to recover from finger pressure, the higher the patient's risk of developing pressure ulcers.

In dark-skinned patients, erythema is hard to discern. Use bright light and look for taut, shiny patches of skin with a purplish tinge. Also, assess carefully for localised heat, induration or oedema, which can be better indicators of ischaemia than erythema.

Category 1 damage: Non-blanchable or persistant erythema

In high-risk patients, non-blanchable tissue can develop in as little as 2 hours. The redness associated with non-blanchable erythema is more intense and doesn't change when compressed with a finger or a clean see-through plastic ruler (or similar). Discoloration of the skin, warmth, oedema, hardness or pain may also be present. Darkly pigmented skin may not have visible blanching. Non-blanchable erythema can be the first sign of tissue destruction. If recognised and treated early, non-blanchable erythema is reversible. The area may be painful, firm, soft, warmer or cooler

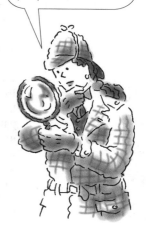

Erythema is often hard to discern in dark-skinned patients. Use a bright light to look for patches of skin that are taut, shiny and purplish in colour.

as compared to adjacent tissue. Category 1 may be difficult to detect in individuals with darker skin tones. It indicates 'at risk' individuals.

Category II: Partial-thickness skin loss or blister

Category II is described as partial-thickness loss of dermis presenting as a shallow open ulcer with a red pink wound bed, without slough. It may also present as an intact or open/ruptured serum or sero sanginous-filled blister. These wounds present as shiny or dry shallow ulcers without slough or bruising. This category should not be used to describe skin tears/tape burns/ epidermal stripping, incontinence associated dermatitis, maceration or excoriation.

Category III: Full-thickness skin loss

In category III ulcers there is full-thickness skin loss. Subcutaneous fat may be visible but bone, tendon or muscle are not exposed or palpable. Some slough may be present and the ulcer may include undermining and tunnelling. The depth of category III pressure ulcers varies by anatomical location. The bridge of the nose, ear, occiput and malleolus do not have (adipose) subcutaneous tissue and category III ulcers in these areas can be shallow. In contrast areas of significant adiposity, extremely deep category III pressure ulcers can develop.

Category IV: Full-thickness tissue loss

Where there is full-thickness tissue loss with exposed bone tendon or muscle, slough or eschar may be present. Often includes undermining and tunnelling, as with category III the depth varies by location. Category IV ulcers can extend into muscle and/or supporting structures (e.g. fascia, tendon or joint capsule) making osteomyelitis or osteitis likely to occur). Exposed bone/muscle is visible or directly palpable.

Additional categories are used in the US.

Full-thickness skin or tissue loss – depth unknown

Full-thickness tissue loss in which the actual depth of the ulcer is completely obscured by slough (yellow, tan, grey, green or brown) and/or eschar (tan, brown or black) in the wound bed. Until the slough and/or eschar are removed to expose the wound bed, the true depth cannot be determined, but it will be either category III or category IV. Stable (dry, adherent, intact without erythema or fluctuance) eschar on the heels serves as 'the body's natural (biological) cover' and should not be removed.

Suspected deep tissue injury (DTI)

Purple or maroon localised area of discoloured intact skin or blood-filled blister due to damage of underlying soft tissue from pressure and/or shear. The discoloured area may be preceded by tissue that is painful, firm, mushy, boggy, warmer or cooler as compared to adjacent tissue. DTI may be difficult to detect in individuals with darker skin tones. Evolution may include a thin blister over a dark wound bed, which evolves to become a thin eschar. Deterioration may be rapid, exposing additional layers of tissue even with treatment.

Size

Carefully trace the wound margins using a grid marked with a cm² grid and a disposable backing sheet. Alternatively, use a disposable measuring tape, measure in cm the wound's length (longest dimension of the wound) and width (longest distance perpendicular to the length). (For further information on measuring size, see Chapter 2, *Dimensions*, page 42.)

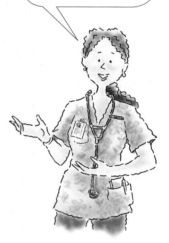

The tissue in the ulcer base may be necrotic, granulation or epithelial tissue.

Depth perception

Measure the ulcer's depth at its deepest point by inserting a gloved finger or a sterile cotton-tipped swab. If you're using a probe other than your finger, be very careful; it's easy to cause further damage. Note any visible tunnels or undermining. If possible, use a gloved finger to gauge the extent.

Base

The type of tissue in the ulcer base determines the potential for healing and the type of treatment used. Know how to identify necrotic, sloughy, granulation and epithelial tissue. (See Chapter 2, *Appearance of wound bed*, page 38.)

Exudate

Exudate is produced as part of the normal process of healing, however, some ulcers with exudate, may take longer to heal. Exudate characteristics include amount, colour, consistency or viscosity and odour. Recording the amount as scant, moderate, large or copious is very subjective, and more frequently now the amount of exudate is quantified by the dressing wear time, for example, dressing needs changing after 3 days. Describe the colour and consistency together with clear, descriptive terms. (See Chapter 2, *Moisture*, page 45.)

The nose knows

Remember all wounds naturally have an odour and some dressing materials produce a distinctive odour. Odour is a subjective observation – one that can suggest a range of things including the presence of infection. It's important to clean the wound thoroughly before assessing the colour and odour of exudate. Otherwise, perceived exudate may be a combination of dressing residue and dead cells – a combination that always produces a noxious odour. (See Chapter 2, *Malodour*, page 46.)

Margins

Pressure ulcer edges have distinct characteristics, including colour, thickness and the degree of attachment to the wound base.

Assess the epithelial rim as an integral part of the wound base. Ideally, there should be a free border of epithelial cells, which proliferate and migrate across the wound bed during healing. When epidermis at the ulcer edges thickens and rolls under, it impairs migration of epithelial cells.

Tunnel troubles

In undermining, which occurs when necrosis of subcutaneous fat or muscle occurs, a pocket extends beneath the skin at the ulcer's edge. Tunnelling differs from undermining in that both ends of a tunnel emerge through the skin's surface. In many cases, a tunnel connects two otherwise distinct pressure ulcers and it may be necessary to open the tunnel before the ulcer(s) can heal.

Sometimes full-thickness pressure ulcers form tracts along fascial planes. When tracts are extensive, external palpation is the only way to determine their direction and length. If this is necessary, use a felt-tipped pen to outline the tract on the skin and measure the resulting image.

Surrounding skin

The skin around the wound should be cleansed at each dressing change to remove dressing residue and exudate and allow visual examination of the skin condition. Assess intact skin surrounding the ulcer for redness, warmth, induration (hardness), swelling and signs of infection. Palpate for heat, pain and oedema. The ulcer bed should be moist but the surrounding skin should be dry. The skin should be adequately moisturised but neither macerated nor eroded. Macerated skin appears waterlogged and may turn white at the wound's edges. Common causes of maceration include wound drainage and urine or faecal contamination. Irritation or stripping may result from poor technique during dressing changes. Skin should also be observed for dryness and cracking (which may indicate the presence of a fungal infection) and also for further damage such as skin stripping, which may be due to use of aggressive adhesives.

Treatment

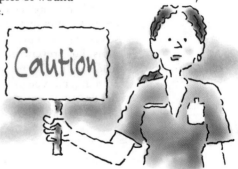

Watch for white, waterlogged skin around the wound's edges. This might indicate maceration.

Caution

Treatment of pressure ulcers follows the basic principles of wound bed preparation plus removal of the cause of damage.
- Debride necrotic tissue and clean the wound to remove debris.
- Provide a moist wound-healing environment through the use of proper dressings.
- Maintain an optimal bacterial balance.
- Protect the wound from further injury.

A key element in all pressure ulcer treatment plans is identifying and treating, when possible, the underlying pathophysiology. If the cause of the ulcer remains, existing ulcers don't heal and new ulcers develop.

Typically, wound care involves cleaning the wound, debriding necrotic tissue and applying a dressing that keeps the wound bed moist. In addition, remember to involve the patient and if appropriate carers, in the care plan to ensure that their objectives are achieved and that they understand their role in the prevention of management of pressure ulcers.

Wound cleaning

Wound cleaning removes wound debris, old dressing materials and necrotic tissue from the wound surface. Whilst saline is frequently used in healthcare settings, water is widely accepted for use in large deep wounds where a large volume of fluid is required, cleansing using a shower hose (if this is not painful) may be a good way of cleaning deep sacral pressure ulcers.

Debridement

Debridement removes non-viable tissue and is the most important factor in wound management. Accurate categorisation and healing can't take place until necrotic tissue is removed. (For more information on debridement, see Chapter 3, page 74.) Remember, sharp debridement should only ever be performed by an appropriately qualified practitioner.

Dressings

Dressings serve to:
- maintain a moist environment
- protect the wound from contamination
- prevent trauma
- provide compression (if bleeding or swelling occurs)
- absorb drainage or debride necrotic tissue.

When choosing a dressing for a pressure ulcer, wound characteristics dictate the type of dressing you use. The dressing selected should protect wound integrity and keep the wound surface moist but prevent an excessive build-up of moisture, which can cause maceration. The frequency of dressing changes depends on the amount and type of wound drainage as well as the characteristics of the dressing.

Wound packing

Wound cavities may require light packing or fill to prevent areas from walling off and developing into abscesses. Remember to be careful with packing because too much packing can generate more pressure and cause additional tissue damage. When absorbent dressings are tightly packed in cavities it limits their ability to absorb.

Patient education

Remember that the goal of patient education is to improve the outcome. For any care plan to succeed after the patient leaves the hospital, they and their carer must understand the care plan, be physically and financially capable of carrying it out at home and value both the information and the outcomes. Therefore, education and goal establishment should take into consideration the preferences and lifestyles of the patient and their family whenever possible.

Get wise to wounds

Pressure ulcer do's and don'ts

With proper skin care and frequent position changes, patients and their carers can keep the patient's skin healthy – a crucial element in pressure ulcer prevention. Here are some important do's and don'ts to pass along to patients:

Do . . .

- Change position at least once every 2 hours while reclining. Follow a schedule. Lie on your right side, then your left side, then your back, then your stomach (if possible). Use pillows and pads for support. Make small turns between the 2-hour changes. Try to use the 30 degree tilt rather than positioning yourself directly on a bone.
- Check your skin for signs of pressure ulcers twice daily. Use a mirror to check areas you can't inspect directly, such as the shoulders, tailbone, hips, elbows, heels and back of the head. Report any breaks in the skin or changes in skin temperature to your nurse.

- Follow the prescribed exercise programme, including range-of-motion exercises every 8 hours or as recommended.
- Eat a well-balanced diet, drink lots of fluids and strive to maintain the recommended weight.
- Use oil-free lotions.

Don't . . .

- Use commercial soaps or skin products that dry or irritate your skin.
- Sleep on wrinkled bed sheets or tuck your covers tightly into the foot of your bed.

Teach the patient and their family how to prevent pressure ulcers and what to do when they occur. (See *Pressure ulcer do's and don'ts*.) Explain repositioning and demonstrate what a 30-degree laterally inclined position looks like. If the patient needs assistance with repositioning, make sure they know the types of devices available and how and where they can be obtained.

Mirror, mirror . . .

Show the patient how to inspect their back and other areas using a mirror. If they can't do this, a family member can help. Make sure they understand the importance of inspecting the skin over bony prominences for pressure-related damage every day.

If the patient needs to apply dressings at home, make sure they know the proper ways to apply and remove them. Ensure that they know how to obtain further dressings and what signs and symptoms should alert them to contact a healthcare professional.

Remember, the goal of patient teaching is to improve the outcome.

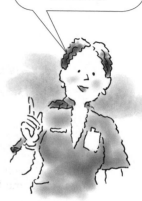

Nag about nutrition

Ensuring proper nutrition can be difficult but the patient and their family need to know how important proper nutrition is to the healing process. Provide materials on nutrition and maintaining an ideal weight, as appropriate. Show the patient how to create an easy-to-read chart of care reminders for home use. If appropriate, refer to a dietician.

In the name of progress

Pressure ulcers should be reassessed weekly. Measure progress by the reduction in necrotic tissue and exudate, and the increase in granulation tissue and epithelial growth as well as changes in size. Remember, pressure ulcers should never be reverse categorised, i.e. they do not go from a category IV to a category III and so on. Clean, well vascularised pressure ulcers should show evidence of healing within 2 weeks. If they don't and the patient has followed the guidelines for nutrition, repositioning, use of support surfaces and wound care, it's time to re-evaluate the care plan.

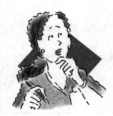

Quick quiz

1. Which body position simultaneously relieves pressure from the sacrum and trochanter?
    A.   prone
    B.   supine
    C.   30-degree lateral position
    D.   90-degree side-lying position.

Answer: C. A 30-degree lateral position is the best way to relieve pressure from both the sacrum and the trochanter at the same time.

2. Which type of wound is created by friction?
    A.   contusion
    B.   laceration
    C.   ulcer
    D.   abrasion.

Answer: D. Abrasions are wounds created by friction.

3. Which serum albumin level would be ranked as moderate?
    A.   2.2 g/dl
    B.   2.5 to 3 g/dl
    C.   3 to 3.5 g/dl
    D.   4 g/dl

Answer: B. A serum albumin level of 2.5 to 3 g/dl is ranked as moderate.

4. Non-blanching erythema is:
   A. red skin which resolves quickly
   B. red skin which does not go white when pressed
   C. red skin which goes white when pressed
   D. white skin which goes red when pressed.

Answer: B. Non-blanching erythema is red skin which does not blanch (go white) with light finger pressure.

5. External factors which increase the risk of pressure damage are:
   A. pressure, shear and friction
   B. pressure, moisture and age
   C. moisture, pressure and diabetes
   D. equipment, age and pressure.

Answer: A. The external factors are pressure, shear and friction.

6. Pressure ulcers can occur in
   A. the elderly
   B. orthopaedics patients
   C. patients with diabetes
   D. any patient group.

Answer: D. Pressure ulcers can occur in any group of patients.

7. Assessing/describing the depth of tissue damage in pressure ulcers is known as:
   A. staging
   B. grading
   C. classification
   D. categorising.

Answer: D. The new guidelines from EPUAP/NPUAP use the term Category of pressure ulcer, i.e. Category I, Category II, Category III and Category IV.

Scoring

★★★ If you answered all seven questions correctly, congratulations! You've certainly demonstrated that you can handle the pressure.

★★ If you answered five or six questions correctly, nicely done! You're near the top of the pressure gradient.

★ If you answered fewer than five questions correctly, don't despair! You'll reposition yourself soon.

References

Bergstrom, N., Braden, B., Kemp, M. *et al.* (1998) Predicting pressure ulcer risk: a multisite study of the predictive validity of the Braden Scale. *Nursing Research* 47(5):261–269.

Elia, M. (2003) *The 'MUST' Report Nutritional Screening for Adults: A Multidisciplinary Responsibility. Development and the use of the 'Malnutrition Universal Screening Tool' (MUST) for Adults.* A report by the Malnutrition Advisory group of the British Association for Parenteral and Enteral Nutrition. Redditch: BAPEN.

European Pressure Ulcer Advisory Panel (EPUAP) (2002) *Summary Report on the Prevalence of Pressure Ulcers EPUAP Review* 4 (2) Accessed on 21/10/08. Available: http://www.epuap.org/review4_2/page8.html

European Pressure Ulcer Advisory Panel (EPUAP) (2003) *Nutritional Guidelines for Pressure Ulcer Prevention and Treatment.* Oxford. EPUAP

European Pressure Ulcer Advisory Panel (EPUAP) (2005) *Pressure Ulcer Classification: Differentiation Between Pressure Ulcers and Moisture Lesions.* Available: http://www.epuap.org/review6_3/page6.html

National Institute of Health and Clinical Excellence (NICE) (2005) *CG029 The Management of Pressure Ulcers in Primary and Secondary Care: A Clinical Practice Guideline* London: RCN

Posnett, J. and Franks, P.J. (2007) The cost of skin breakdown and ulceration in the UK In: *Skin Breakdown the Silent Epidemic.* Hull: Smith and Nephew Foundation.

Waterlow, J. (2005) From costly treatment to cost-effective prevention: using Waterlow. *British Journal of Community Nursing (Wound Care suppl)* 10(9):S25–S30.

9 Diabetic foot ulcers

Just the facts

In this chapter, you'll learn:

♦ causes of diabetic foot ulcers
♦ prevention measures for diabetic foot ulcers
♦ assessment criteria for diabetic foot ulcers
♦ interventions for diabetic foot ulcer treatment.

A look at diabetic foot ulcers

Diabetes mellitus is a metabolic disorder characterised by hyperglycaemia resulting from lack of insulin, lack of insulin effect or both. Insulin transports glucose into cells, where it's used as fuel or stored as glycogen. Insulin also stimulates protein synthesis and storage of free fatty acids in fat deposits. An insulin deficiency compromises these important functions. Diabetes can begin suddenly or develop insidiously. (See *Diabetes: The not-so-sweet facts*, page 198.)

High plasma glucose levels caused by diabetes can damage blood vessels and nerves. Therefore, patients with diabetes are prone to developing foot ulcers due to nerve damage and poor circulation to the lower extremities. One in seven diabetic patients will develop a foot ulcer in their lifetime (Reiber 2001). These ulcers are hard to heal and can result in infection, extensive tissue damage, amputation and long-term disability (Edmonds 2007). Good diabetes control and attention to foot care can help prevent these problems developing or at least make them less serious.

Causes

Diabetic neuropathy, pressure and other mechanical forces and PVD can cause foot ulcers in patients with diabetes.

197

Diabetes: The not-so-sweet facts

Diabetes has been characterised as a modern day epidemic and it isn't hard to understand why when you look at the statistics for the UK.

Prevalence

There are an estimated 2.35 million people with diabetes in England alone. This is predicted to grow to more than 2.5 million by 2010; 9% of this figure will be due to an increase in obesity (DoH 2007).

Amputations

Amongst people who have diabetes, amputations are reported to be 15 times more common than amongst other people. Fifty per cent of all amputations occur in people who have diabetes. (Diabetes.co.uk, 2008) and 85% of amputations are preceded by an ulcer (Pecoraro *et al.* 1990).

Cost

Around 5 per cent of total NHS spend (and up to 10 per cent of hospital in-patient spend) is used for the care of people with diabetes (DoH 2007).

Mortality

Mortality attributed to people with diabetes is suggested as 4.2% of deaths in men and 7.7% of deaths in women in the UK (NICE 2008).

Diabetic neuropathy

Peripheral neuropathy is the primary cause of diabetic foot ulcer development. Neuropathy is a nerve disorder that results in impaired or lost function in the tissues served by the affected nerve fibres. In diabetes, neuropathy may be caused by ischaemia due to thickening in the tiny blood vessels that supply the nerve or by nerve demyelinisation (destruction of the protective myelin sheath surrounding a nerve), which slows the conduction of impulses.

Polyneuropathy, or damage to multiple types of nerves, is the most common form of neuropathy

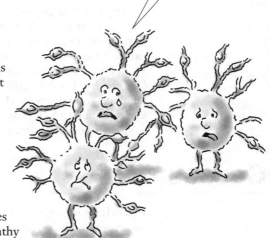

How tri-ing! The trineuropathy that commonly develops in the feet of diabetic patients includes loss of sensation, motor function and autonomic function.

in patients with diabetes. In the foot, a trineuropathy develops that includes:

- loss of sensation
- loss of motor function
- loss of autonomic functions (the autonomic nervous system controls smooth muscles, glands and visceral organs).

(See *Understanding diabetic trineuropathy*, page 200.)

Typically, impairment affects the feet and hands first and then progresses towards the knees and elbows, respectively. This presentation is called a stocking and glove distribution.

No more warnings!

As sensory nerves degenerate and die (sensory neuropathy), the patient experiences a burning or 'pins-and-needles' sensation that might worsen at night.

As sensation declines, the patient risks foot injury. Impaired sensation prevents the patient from feeling stimuli, such as pain and pressure, which normally warn of impending damage. Anything from stepping on something sharp to wearing ill-fitting shoes can result in foot injury because the patient can't feel the damage happening.

A trophy that isn't a prize

As motor nerves degenerate and die (motor neuropathy), muscles in the limbs atrophy, especially the intrinsic muscles of the feet, which causes footdrop and structural deformities. These degenerative changes increase the patient's risk of stumbling or falling and further damaging the foot.

Infection alert

As autonomic nerves degenerate and die (autonomic neuropathy), sweat and sebaceous glands malfunction and skin on the patient's feet dries and cracks. If fissures develop, bacteria can gain entry and the risk of infection rises. Also, the inhibition of resident skin bacteria can be affected by reduced sebum production and by the decreased immune response associated with diabetes (Robbins 2007). When the growth of these 'good' bacteria is inhibited, fungal infections such as tinea pedis (athlete's foot) can flourish.

Mechanical forces

Mechanical forces that can cause diabetic foot ulcers include pressure, friction and shear.

Understanding diabetic trineuropathy

Uncontrolled diabetes commonly results in a trineuropathy (three concurrent neuropathies) that dramatically increases a patient's risk of developing diabetic foot ulcers.

Sensory neuropathy

In sensory neuropathy, ischaemia or demyelinisation (see illustration below) causes nerve death or deterioration. When this occurs, the patient no longer feels painful stimuli and can't respond appropriately.

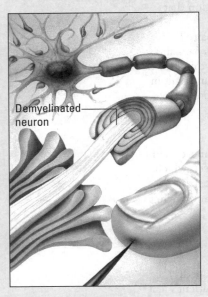

Demyelinated neuron

Motor neuropathy

In motor neuropathy, intrinsic muscles deep in the plantar surface of the foot atrophy, resulting in increased arch height and clawed toes. In addition, the fat pad that normally covers the metatarsal heads migrates towards the toes, exposing the metatarsal heads to more pressure and increasing pressure ulcer risk. The risk of ulcer development is high for the upper surfaces of clawed toes as well, especially if the patient has poorly fitted shoes.

The illustration below shows the degenerative changes in the foot resulting from motor neuropathy. Shading indicates the areas where ulcers are most likely to develop.

Increased arch height

Clawed toes

Downward displacement of the metatarsal heads (with loss of fat pad)

Autonomic neuropathy

In uncontrolled diabetes, autonomic neuropathy inhibits or destroys the sympathetic component of the autonomic nervous system, which controls vasoconstriction in peripheral blood vessels. The resulting unfettered flow of blood to the lower limbs and feet may cause osteopenia (reduction of bone volume) in foot and ankle bones.

In Charcot's disease (neuropathic osteoarthropathy), bones weakened by osteopenia suffer fractures that the patient doesn't feel due to sensory neuropathy. Over time, this process causes bony dissolution that culminates with the collapse of the midfoot into a rocker bottom deformity (see illustration below). Patients with Charcot's disease are placed on non-weight-bearing status until inflammation subsides.

Midfoot ulcers resulting from increased plantar pressures over the rocker bottom deformity heal slower than ulcers on the forefoot.

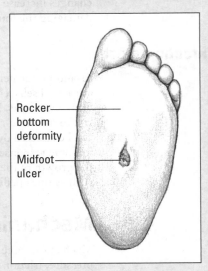

Rocker bottom deformity

Midfoot ulcer

Pressure

Sensory neuropathy places a patient at increased risk for diabetic foot ulcers caused by pressure – especially a patient who's confined to a bed or wheelchair. Such a patient can suffer damage simply by letting his feet rest for too long on a bed or a wheelchair footrest. Impaired sensation prevents the patient from feeling the discomfort that results from staying in one position too long.

Prominent plantar pressure places

As with pressure ulcers, areas over bony prominences are the most common places for diabetic foot ulcers, including:
- metatarsal heads
- great toe
- the heel.

Friction and shear

Although pressure is the major mechanical force at work in the development of diabetic ulcers, it isn't the only one. Friction and shear can cause damage as well. A loose shoe rubbing against the foot or a foot sliding across a bed sheet can cause friction damage.

Shearly it's true

Shearing forces build up when damp skin sticks to a surface while the underlying bone and tissue move. For example, the skin of a sweating foot can cling to a shoe while the underlying tissues slide beneath the skin.

Peripheral vascular disease

A common problem in patients with diabetes, PVD impairs the healing process of existing ulcers and may contribute to neuropathy as well. In PVD, atherosclerosis narrows the peripheral arteries, slowly reducing the flow of blood to the limbs. (See *How atherosclerosis impairs circulation*, page 202.) As perfusion decreases, the risks of ischaemia and tissue necrosis increase.

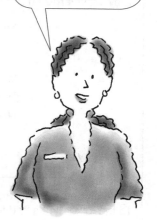

Remember that, along with pressure, friction and shear can also cause diabetic ulcers.

Risk factors

Identifying the patient's risk factors is an important part of prevention. Loss of sensation is the single biggest risk factor but it isn't the only one. Here's a list of general risk factors for diabetic ulcers:
- structural foot deformity (such as clawed toes, rocker bottom or hallux vagus)
- trauma and improperly fitted shoes

How atherosclerosis impairs circulation

In atherosclerosis, fatty deposits (cholesterol) and fibrous plaques accumulate along the walls of the arteries, narrowing the lumen and reducing the artery's elasticity. Thrombi (blood clots) form on the roughened surface of plaques and may grow large enough to block the artery's lumen.

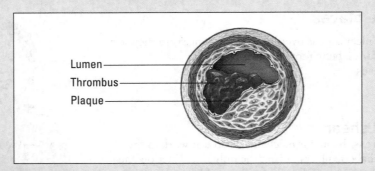

Lumen
Thrombus
Plaque

In diabetes, the arterial damage caused by atherosclerosis reduces blood flow to the lower limbs and to the nerves that innervate them. In addition to promoting ulcer development, poor perfusion slows the healing process for existing ulcers and impedes circulation of systemic antibiotics to infected areas.

- calluses
- prolonged, elevated pressure on areas of tissue
- limited joint mobility
- prolonged history of diabetes
- blindness or partial sight
- chronic renal disease.

Risk factors for diabetic foot ulcers may also be either local or systemic. Local risk factors include:
- previous foot ulcer or amputation
- neuropathy
- PVD.

Systemic risk factors include:
- age (older than age 65)
- hypertension
- hyperglycaemia
- hyperlipidaemia
- obesity

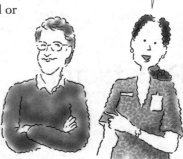

Teaching your patients how to eliminate or minimise diabetic ulcer risk factors is the best form of prevention.

Prevention

Diabetic ulcer prevention starts with identifying the patient's risk factors and then teaching him how to eliminate or minimise these risks.

Patient teaching

Patient education and involvement is an integral part of diabetes management. Teach the patient about ulcer care and prevention and the importance of controlling diabetes, including the consequences of not controlling it – for example, teach him that poorly controlled blood glucose levels can lead to peripheral neuropathy and vascular damage. Research indicates that tight glycaemic control reduces the frequency and severity of neuropathy in patients with type 1 and 2 diabetes (NICE 2007a, NICE 2008). Teach the patient proper foot care and steps they can take to prevent ulcers, including daily examinations, skin washing and maintenance techniques, toenail care and exercise. Also instruct them on how to choose proper socks and shoes. (See *Proper foot care*, page 204.)

A clean sock a day keeps the doctor away

White cotton-blended socks are the best choice for a patient with diabetes. Cotton-blended socks wick away moisture and allow air to circulate around the foot. White socks vividly show blood or exudate from an injury or ulcer that the patient may not feel. Regardless of the material, socks should always be non-constricting and seamless over bony prominences. Socks with added padding can provide additional cushioning as well as some protection from shearing force.

Team effort

Successful prevention programmes for diabetic ulcers begin with health promotion. In the UK, NICE guidance (NICE 2007b) states that all patients with diabetes should have an annual review which should include a foot examination for risk of ulceration. Care of people at low risk of ulceration (normal sensation and palpable pulses) should include a foot care management plan and education. People at increased risk (neuropathy, absent pulses or other risk factor) should have a 3–6 month review by the foot protection team. People at high risk (neuropathy, absent pulses or other risk

Fancy footwork

Proper foot care

Here are some tips to teach your patient to help ensure proper foot care.

Performing foot hygiene

- Check your feet daily for injury or pressure areas (a long-handled mirror can help).
- Wash your feet with a mild soap and dry thoroughly between your toes.
- Check your bath water to make sure it isn't too hot (test the water with a thermometer or ask a family member to help).
- Apply a moisturising cream to prevent dry, cracking skin on your feet and to balance skin pH. Don't apply moisturiser between the toes.
- Cut your toenails off squarely; see a podiatrist if they're dystrophic (deformed and thickened).
- Don't go barefooted – the risk of injury is too great.

Choosing socks

- Use silver ion-lined socks for fungus control.
- Wear white or light-coloured socks in order to quickly detect bleeding from trauma.
- Wear natural fibre socks because they breathe better than synthetics.
- Wear socks that wick perspiration away from your feet (such as cotton-blended socks) to prevent maceration.
- Use diabetic padded socks for shear and friction control.

Choosing shoes

- Wear well-fitting shoes, not shoes that are too tight or loose.
- Wear shoes that breathe to reduce maceration and fungal infections.
- Wear new shoes for short periods (under 1 hour) each day initially; gradually increase the time as your feet adjust.
- If you have any foot deformities or a history of ulceration, wear professionally fitted shoes.
- Wash your shoes, if possible, to destroy microorganisms.
- Check your shoes before putting them on to make sure nothing has fallen in which could cause harm.

factor plus foot deformity, skin changes or previous ulcer) should have a 1–3 monthly review by the foot protection team. Diabetics presenting with a foot care emergency (swelling, new ulcer, discoloration) should be referred to a multiprofessional diabetic foot care team within 24 hours.

The patient should play an active role in setting personal healthcare goals, working in partnership with the healthcare team to achieve those goals.

Most patients with diabetes have multiple disorders, requiring a series of interventions involving many health disciplines – nurses, doctors, physiotherapists, occupational therapists, dietitians, podiatrists, endocrinologists, psychologists, diabetes educators, prosthetists or orthotists and social workers.

Assessment

Assessment of diabetic foot ulcers includes gathering a thorough patient history and performing a physical examination and special testing of the lower extremities.

History

A thorough patient history is the key to assessing diabetic foot ulcers. In addition to the basic information elicited during a traditional patient history, ask the patient about:
- date of onset of diabetes
- management measures
- glycaemic control (using the glycosylated haemoglobin level as an indicator)
- medications
- other diagnosed problems (especially hypertriglyceridaemia)
- status and history of any diagnosed neuropathy
- allergies, especially skin reactions
- tobacco and alcohol use
- recent changes in activity level
- date and location of previous ulcerations
- date that they first noticed the current ulcer
- the way in which the ulcer occurred
- type and quality of any associated pain
- their level of knowledge and understanding.

Physical examination

Use a holistic approach when performing the assessment, which consists of a general examination and an examination of the patient's feet. Remember that the patient's overall physical health and state of mind affect wound healing.

General examination

During the general assessment, you will need to evaluate the patient's musculoskeletal, neurological, vascular and integumentary systems to provide perspective for assessing the condition of their lower limbs.

Bone up

Assess these aspects of the patient's musculoskeletal system:
- posture
- gait

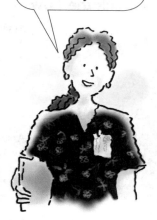

Treat the body as a unit, and remember, a thorough assessment of the patient's condition requires examination of several systems.

- strength, flexibility and endurance
- range of motion.

Make connections

Assess these aspects of the patient's neurological system:
- balance
- reflexes
- sensory function.

Check the flow

Assess these aspects of the patient's vascular system:
- posterior tibial and dorsalis pedis pulses
- ankle–brachial pressure index (ABPI).
  Keep in mind that ABPI isn't as reliable due to calcification in the microvasculature.

Skin deep

Assess these aspects of the patient's integumentary system:
- texture
- temperature
- colour
- appendages (hair, sweat glands, sebaceous glands, nails).

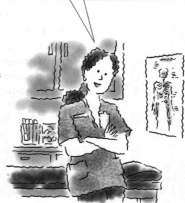

Be sure to check the high-risk areas of your patient's feet for evidence of ulcers.

Foot examination

Carefully examine the patient's feet to detect and assess foot ulcers. Check the following high-risk areas of the feet for existing or impending ulcers (calluses, for example):
- plantar surfaces (soles) of the toes
- tips of the toes
- area between the toes (look for athlete's foot or *tinea pedis*)
- lateral aspect of the foot's plantar surface.
  Wound characteristics depend on where the wound occurs on the foot. (See *Features of diabetic foot ulcers*, page 207.) Characteristics of surrounding skin may include:
- calluses (considered pre-wounds)
- blood blisters (haemorrhage beneath a callus)
- erythema (a sign of inflammation or infection)
- induration (hardened edges)
- skin fissures (portals for bacterial entry)
- dry, scaly skin.

Special testing

Special tests provide a clearer picture of lower leg and foot health. These tests evaluate pressure, neurological function and perfusion.

Features of diabetic foot ulcers

In diabetic foot ulcers, characteristic clinical features depend on the ulcer's location.

Ulcer location	Clinical features
Plantar surface	Even wound margins
Great toe	Deep wound bed
Metatarsal head	Dry or low-to-moderate exudate
Heel	Low-to-moderate exudate
Tip or top of toe	Pale granulation with ischaemia or bright-red, friable granulation tissue with infection

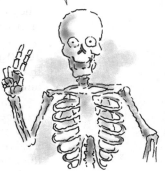

Harris mat prints and computerised pressure mapping are musculoskeletal tests that can aid you when assessing plantar pressures.

The results provide insight into the mechanism of injury, condition of the wound bed and surrounding tissue, prognosis for healing and required treatment interventions.

Musculoskeletal tests

Harris mat prints and computerised pressure mapping are special musculoskeletal tests that provide information about the plantar pressures of the foot.

Harris mat prints

Pressure over bony prominences is one cause of diabetic foot ulcers. A simple method for determining areas of increased pressure on the plantar surface of the foot is to use an ink mat.

Making an impression

In Harris mat prints, the examiner inks the bottom of the mat, which has a grid to aid assessment of results, and places it on an evaluation template or clean sheet of paper. Then the patient steps on the uninked top surface of the mat, placing equal weight on each foot. If needed, the examiner holds the patient's outstretched hands to help ensure equal weight distribution. The impression on the template or sheet of paper shows relative areas of pressure under the patient's foot. Darker areas on the grid indicate high-pressure areas. In a case where a dynamic impression is required, the patient slowly walks across the mat to create the impression.

Under pressure

High-pressure areas usually correlate with calluses (pre-wounds) or existing wounds. The results help guide the choice of special off-loading devices, which help relieve pressure when the patient stands or walks.

Computerised pressure mapping

Computerised pressure mapping devices test plantar pressures while the patient is wearing a shoe and when he's barefoot. The approach is similar to Harris mat prints; however, in this test, a computer maps the pressures and displays the results on a printout. A colour gradient illustrates relative pressure, with red and orange indicating areas where pressure is highest.

Neurological tests

Neurological tests for the lower extremities include deep tendon reflexes testing, vibration perception testing with a tuning fork or biothesiometer and 10 g monofilament testing for protective sensation.

Deep tendon reflexes testing

Peripheral neuropathy causes a decrease in deep tendon reflexes. Decreased deep tendon reflexes correlate with muscular atrophy, usually the intrinsic muscles of the foot in a patient with diabetes. The assessor uses the pointed end of a reflex hammer to strike the biceps, triceps, brachioradialis, patellar and Achilles reflexes.

Tuning fork test

In this test, the assessor uses a tuning fork to assess peripheral nerve function and help identify and quantify existing neuropathy.

Tuning up
* The examiner activates the tuning fork and holds it against a bony prominence in the affected limb (for example, a metatarsal head or malleoli) and then records the patient's ability to sense the vibration.
* Next, the examiner tests other bony prominences in the body (for example, the patella or elbow) or the same prominence in the opposite limb if it's unaffected.
* Afterwards, the results are compared to assess neurological function.

Biothesiometer

A biothesiometer is another tool that's used to assess the patient's vibratory perception threshold. It provides a better quantitative measurement of vibratory sense than the tuning fork. Patients with sensory neuropathy have impaired vibratory perception thresholds (less than 25 volts, as measured on the biothesiometer).

10 g monofilament test

The 10 g monofilament test helps determine the level of protective sensation in the feet. While the patient's eyes are closed, the

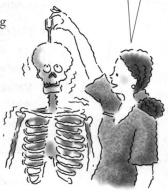

Just relax and focus on good vibrations, O.K.?

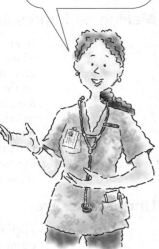

When performing the 10 g monofilament test, you'll use a monofilament to test the patient's level of protective sensation in his feet.

Performing a 10 g monofilament test

In this test, the examiner uses a 10 g monofilament to assess protective sensation in the patient's feet. This illustration shows the points to test.

How it's done

The examiner places the 10-g monofilament on one of the testing points and exerts enough pressure to bow the monofilament (as illustrated). With their eyes closed, the patient must then identify where and when they feel the monofilament touch.

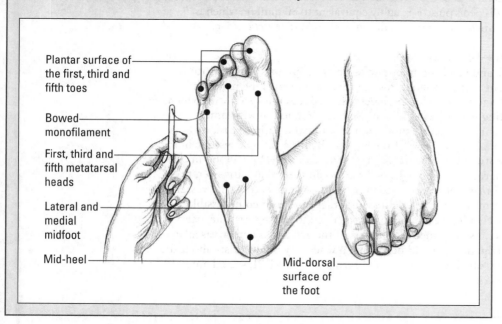

Plantar surface of the first, third and fifth toes

Bowed monofilament

First, third and fifth metatarsal heads

Lateral and medial midfoot

Mid-heel

Mid-dorsal surface of the foot

examiner holds a 10 g monofilament perpendicular to the patient's foot and then presses the monofilament against the skin until it bows. The patient is then asked to identify when and where the skin has been touched. As protective sensation decreases, plantar pressures tend to rise, as does the patient's risk of ulcers at these points. (See *Performing the 10 g monofilament test*.)

Vascular tests

Vascular tests help assess circulation in the lower extremities. These tests include pulse palpation, ABPI, measuring toe pressures and obtaining transcutaneous oxygen ($TcPO_2$) levels.

Pulse palpation

Initial assessment of limb perfusion includes palpating the dorsalis pedis, posterior tibial, popliteal and femoral pulses. If it's hard to palpate a pulse due to oedema, consider using Doppler ultrasound, which produces an audible signal coinciding with the pulse.

Hear the beat

Hold the transducer at a 45-degree angle to the skin, towards the direction of blood flow and listen for the beats. The results provide a general idea of the circulation to each level of the limb. A palpable dorsalis pedis pulse is roughly equivalent to 80 mmHg, which is adequate for healing most diabetic wounds. (See *Pulse rating*.)

Ankle–brachial index

PVD and resulting poor perfusion are common problems for patients with diabetes. Poor perfusion increases the patient's likelihood of developing ulcers and reduces the speed with which existing ulcers heal. ABPI is used in conjunction with other vascular tests to determine and monitor the patient's risk of ischaemia in the area of the ankle. ABPI is a ratio of systolic blood pressure in the brachial artery in the arm to systolic blood pressure measured in the dorsalis pedis artery in the ankle. However, the ABPI may not be accurate in patients with diabetes if the vessels being measured are calcified and, therefore, not compressible. A falsely high reading may be seen due to incompressible artery walls caused by medial sclerosis of the arteries. Further vascular investigations should be arranged when any doubt exists about the results obtained. (For more information on ABPI, see Chapter 10, *Leg Ulcers*.)

Pulse rating

When assessing the amplitude of a pulse, rate the strength on a numeric scale, such as the one below.

Rating	Pulse characteristic
0	No palpable pulse
+1	Weak or thready pulse: hard to feel, easily obliterated by slight finger pressure
+2	Normal pulse: easily palpable, obliterated by strong finger pressure
+3	Bounding pulse: readily palpable, forceful, not easily obliterated by finger pressure

Toe pressures

Toe pressures may be a more sensitive indicator of changes in vascular integrity in the distal areas of the foot. Toe pressures are performed in the same manner as limb blood pressures, except that a much smaller, specialised cuff is used for the toe. Due to the tiny arteries in digits, the corresponding arterial pressures are lower than those measured in an arm or a leg. Typical pressure in the toe is about 70% of systolic values obtained in the arm.

The toes have it

A toe pressure of 45 mmHg or higher is needed for healing to occur. Toe pressures allow you to gauge the patient's ischaemic risk profile. Generally, a toe pressure:
- above 55 mmHg reflects a low risk of tissue ischaemia
- below 40 mmHg reflects a high risk of ischaemia
- below 20 mmHg reflects a severe risk of ischaemia.

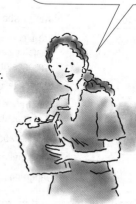

Your patient needs a toe pressure of 45 mmHg or higher in order to heal.

Transcutaneous oxygen levels

A $TcPO_2$ of 30% or higher is required for healing. $TcPO_2$ levels reflect the oxygen saturation of tissues. Typically, $TcPO_2$ levels are measured close to the ulcer. In general, a $TcPO_2$ level:
- above 40% reflects a low risk of tissue ischaemia
- between 20% and 30% reflects a high risk of ischaemia
- below 20% reflects a severe risk of ischaemia.

Classification

Diabetic foot ulcers are classified according to depth, presence of ischaemia and presence of infection, depending on the classification system. The Wagner Ulcer Grade Classification (Wagner 1981) and the University of Texas Diabetic Foot Classification System (Lavery *et al.* 1997) are two commonly used classification systems.

Wagner Ulcer Grade Classification

The original Wagner Ulcer Grade Classification considers depth of penetration; however, it doesn't allow for the assessment of infection at all tissue levels. A modified version of the Wagner classification system adds levels to take into account infection and ischaemia. (See *Wagner Ulcer Grade Classification*, page 212.)

Wagner Ulcer Grade Classification

In the Wagner Ulcer Grade Classification, less complex ulcers receive lower scores; more complex ulcers, higher scores. Ulcers with higher scores may require surgical intervention or amputation.

Grade	Characteristics
0	• Pre-ulcer lesion • Healed ulcer • Presence of bony deformity
1	• Superficial ulcer without subcutaneous tissue involvement
2	• Penetration through the subcutaneous tissue; may expose bone, tendon, ligament or joint capsule
3	• Osteitis, abscess or osteomyelitis
4	• Gangrene of a digit
5	• Gangrene requiring foot amputation

Adapted with permission from Wagner, F.W., Jr. The diabetic foot. *Orthopedics* 10:163–172, 1987. © Slack Incorporated.

University of Texas Diabetic Foot Classification System

The University of Texas Diabetic Foot Classification System takes tissue infection and ischaemia into consideration and provides a more detailed breakdown of classifications than the Wagner system. (See *University of Texas Diabetic Foot Classification System*, page 213.)

Complications

The most common complication that impedes the healing of diabetic foot ulcers and can cause a wound to become chronic is infection. Other complications include:
• multiple comorbidities, including PVD, which cause a number of problems that increase the risk of ulceration and reduce the likelihood of speedy healing

University of Texas Diabetic Foot Classification System

The University of Texas Diabetic Foot Classification System provides a detailed categorisation of diabetic foot ulcers. Staging the ulcer from A to D is a predictor of amputation (stage D is at greatest risk) and grading it from 0 to III is an indicator of infection (grade III is at greatest risk).

Stage	Grade 0	Grade I	Grade II	Grade III
A	Pre-ulcerative or post-ulcerative foot at risk for further ulceration	Superficial ulcer without tendon, capsule or bone involvement	Ulcer penetrating to tendon or joint capsule	Ulcer penetrating to bone
B	Presence of infection	Presence of infection	Presence of infection	Presence of infection
C	Presence of ischaemia	Presence of ischaemia	Presence of ischaemia	Presence of ischaemia
D	Presence of infection and ischaemia	Presence of infection and ischaemia	Presence of infection and ischaemia	Presence of infection and ischaemia

Adapted with permission from Armstrong, D.G., *et al.* Treatment-based classification system for assessment and care of diabetic feet. *JAPMA* 86(7):311–316, 1996.

• uncontrolled hyperglycaemia, which commonly signals infection and inhibits the immune system, particularly the scavenging function of neutrophils
• psychosocial problems, such as depression and poverty, which profoundly affect the patient's nutritional status, in turn affecting the body's ability to prevent ulcers and heal existing wounds.

Infection

An infection in the wound or elsewhere consumes protein needed for healing and interferes directly by damaging the wound bed. Infections fall into two categories: non-limb-threatening or limb-threatening. Non-limb-threatening infections tend to be superficial infections involving tissues within 2 cm of the wound margin. In this type of infection, no significant tissue ischaemia is present and bone isn't palpable in the wound bed. Non-limb-threatening infection can be treated with topical antimicrobials, sharp debridement by a suitably qualified practitioner and wound cleaning once or twice daily.

In contrast, limb-threatening infection involves tissue more than 2 cm from the wound margin, palpable bone in the wound bed and tissue ischaemia. When this occurs, hospitalisation and surgical debridement of infected bone and soft tissues are

> Comorbidities are speed bumps on the remedial road. They can slow healing of existing ulcers and contribute to new ones.

necessary. Unless the infected bone is fully resected, the patient may require 4 to 8 weeks of I.V. antibiotic therapy.

Show me a sign

Uncontrollable blood glucose or hyperglycaemia may be the first sign of infection because patients with diabetes commonly fail to demonstrate the typical systemic responses. A 4° to 5° difference in temperature between similar areas on each foot is a local sign of infection. An infrared scanner thermometer is the most reliable way to check this difference. An infection in the wound bed commonly causes friable (easy to bleed), bright-red granulation tissue.

Deep trouble

Osteomyelitis or bone infection is common in deep wounds. A quick and reliable method for determining whether osteomyelitis is present in a diabetic ulcer bed is to palpate for bone. A palpable bone usually indicates osteomyelitis; however, osteomyelitis may be difficult to distinguish from acute Charcot's neuropathic osteoarthropathy. The best way to differentiate between the two is to culture a bone fragment from the wound bed, however this is invasive and a non-invasive imaging technique (MRI) should be used in preference where possible.

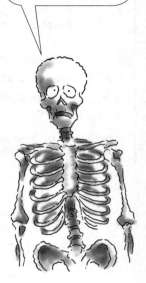

If you palpate bone in a diabetic ulcer bed, your patient probably has osteomyelitis. Culture a bone fragment to make sure.

Treatment

Successful healing depends on proper wound cleaning and dressing and off-loading. Topical antimicrobials, debridement, biotherapies and surgery may also be included in the care plan.

Wound cleaning

Wound cleaning is a fundamental step in the healing process because necrotic tissue is a reservoir for bacteria and inhibits wound healing.

Flushing the wound bed with normal saline (0.9%) is the best method of cleaning a diabetic foot ulcer. Commercial wound cleaners can be toxic to cells in the wound bed; thus, their use can slow healing. Use clean, warm water and aqueous cream to clean the surrounding skin. Dry thoroughly but carefully.

Dressings

Moist (not wet) wound therapy speeds healing in diabetic foot ulcers. Dressings that maintain the necessary moist wound environment include:
- alginates
- hydrofibres
- foams
- hydrocolloids
- hydrogels (with caution)
- composites (combinations of dressings)
- antimicrobials.

Wise choice

The dressing you choose depends on the condition of your patient's ulcer. Diabetic foot ulcers tend to produce low-to-moderate drainage; however, if the wound bed is dry, it needs a dressing that adds moisture. Either amorphous hydrogels or sheet hydrogels can help in this case. Hydrogel sheets are more cost-effective but don't work as well in deeper wounds. For deep or tunnelling ulcers that require gentle packing, hydrogel-impregnated gauze is a less costly alternative to amorphous hydrogels. All hydrogel dressings add moisture to the wound bed because they're made up of as much as 95% water. Hydrogels also encourage autolytic debridement but be cautious as hydrogels, if overused, will cause maceration to the skin surrounding the ulcer and possibly further skin breakdown. Hydroclloids should also be used with caution in diabetic foot ulceration. If the wound requires regular reassessment (diabetic ulcers can deteriorate very quickly), the frequent application and removal of a hydrocolloid dressing (which is adhesive) may cause skin trauma. In addition, hydrocolloids are designed to stay in place for several days for optimal effect and frequent renewal will be both expensive and clinically ineffective. (See *Dressings for diabetic foot ulcers*, page 216.)

> Relieving pressure from plantar surfaces – known as *off-loading* – is key to pressure ulcer treatment and prevention.

Off-loading

Off-loading (relieving pressure) plantar tissues is the cornerstone of diabetic neuropathy treatment as well as prevention for those patients at risk for recurrent breakdown. Off-loading seeks to control, limit or remove all intrinsic and extrinsic factors that increase plantar pressures. Examples of intrinsic risk factors include faulty biomechanics in the foot or the presence of a bony deformity. Extrinsic risk factors

Dress for success

Dressings for diabetic foot ulcers

Use this chart to help you choose an appropriate dressing for your patient's foot ulcer.

Type of ulcer	Recommended dressings
Dry	• Hydrogel (with caution not to overuse)
Wet	• Alginate • Foam • Hydrofibre
Necrotic	• Hydrogel • Hydrocolloid
Shallow	• Foam • Hydrocolloid
Tunnelling or deep	• Alginate ropes or hydrofibres (for wet ulcers) • Hydrogel-impregnated gauze (for dry ulcers)
Infected	• Antimicrobial e.g. Iodosorb (a gel that cleans the wound by absorbing fluid, exudate and bacteria)
Bleeding	• Alginate • Hydrofibre

include trauma, ill-fitting shoes or maintaining a position for too long, which allows for the buildup of damaging pressure.

Damage control

Because patients with diabetic neuropathy can no longer feel the growing discomfort that precedes tissue damage, off-loading is particularly important. Both non-surgical and surgical off-loading interventions help prevent or limit the kind of tissue damage that causes ulcers to form.

Non-surgical off-loading interventions

Non-surgical interventions include therapeutic footwear, custom orthotics and walking casts. When considering a device, keep in mind that using a device can increase the patient's risk of falling. Be sure to provide instructions on fall prevention.

Therapeutic footwear

A patient with recurring ulcers and severe foot deformities can greatly benefit from a custom-moulded shoe. Common design

Therapeutic shoe modifications

These illustrations show the modifications in custom shoes that can improve stability and accommodate the deformities that affect many patients with diabetes.

High top

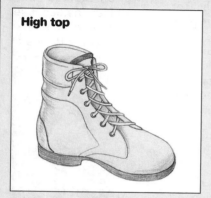

Lateral flare

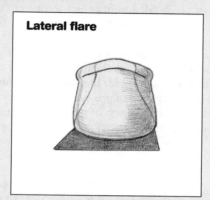

Rocker sole

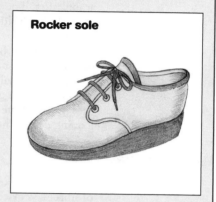

features of therapeutic footwear include:
- soft, breathable leather that conforms to foot deformities
- high tops for ankle stability
- rocker soles and bottoms for pressure and pain relief across the plantar metatarsal heads
- a toe box with extra depth and width to accommodate deformities, such as clawed toes and hallux valgus (displacement of the great toe towards the other toes)
- flared lateral soles for stability. (See *Therapeutic shoe modifications*.)

Custom orthotics

Custom orthotics are shoe inserts that serve various functions based on the patient's needs. In general, custom orthotics relieve pressure, reduce shearing force and friction, and cushion the foot against shocks. If necessary, custom orthotics accommodate the patient's foot deformities as well.

Walking casts

Walking casts range from total contact casts to splints and walkers.

Cast member

A total contact cast is the top of the line in care for uninfected diabetic ulcers on the plantar surface of the foot. Total contact casts are custom made for each patient by a healthcare professional, typically an orthotist or surgical appliances officer. Inside the cast, padding is fitted over bony areas of the ankle and leg that are at risk for pressure ulcers. A plaster shell reinforced with plaster splints covers the padding. Fibreglass covers the plaster to lend rigidity and additional strength, and the cast includes a sturdy walking heel for ambulation. The cast is moulded to fit snugly to prevent the foot from sliding inside it. This reduces shearing forces over the plantar surface.

A patient with an infected diabetic ulcer isn't a candidate for a total contact cast because a cast makes daily assessment, cleaning and antimicrobial therapy impossible. In addition, inflammation and oedema can cause a build-up of pressure within the cast and subsequent tissue damage. In the case of infection, a removable off-loading device should be used.

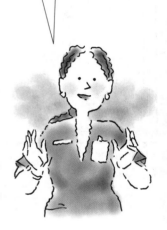

A total contact cast is out of the question for a patient with an infected foot ulcer. Instead, use a removable off-loading device.

Walk this way

Splints and walkers have cushioned inserts with an outer shell of fibreglass or copolymer. Several splint and walker options are available. One advantage of splints and walkers is that they allow easy inspection of the ulcer. In addition, off-loading modifications can be accomplished relatively easily by changing the type of splint or walker in use. However, these devices have disadvantages as well. First and foremost, they don't provide the same degree of pressure and shear relief as a total contact cast. Also, for these therapies to work, the patient must be committed to using the device – a patient can always take a splint off or choose not to use a walker.

Surgical off-loading interventions

Surgical off-loading procedures include surgical dissection of the wound bed and pressure-inducing bony tissue deformities. Pressure over bony prominences compresses and occludes blood vessels, causing ischaemia. Resection (surgical removal) of bony deformities reduces peak plantar pressures. This type of surgery is called curative surgery because it removes the pathological tissue. Examples of curative surgery include exostectomy, digital arthroplasty, bone and joint resections and partial calcanectomy.

Topical antimicrobials

Applying a topical antimicrobial directly to the wound bed can help control microorganisms in the wound bed and improve healing. The most frequently used ones in modern wound care include those containing iodine or silver, which kills or inhibits microbes. The active ingredients are released slowly in concentrations that are toxic to microbes but not to important cells in the wound bed such as fibroblasts. Topical antimicrobial agents usually have a non-specific mode of action so the opportunity exists for unwanted patient effects, but the chance of developing resistance in microbial species is lessened (Cooper 2004). It remains important to be cautious when using antimicrobial dressings as links between antiseptic and antibiotic resistance have been reported.

Debridement

Debriding necrotic and non-viable tissue, foreign matter and microbes from the wound bed expedites wound healing. The most effective method of debridement, surgical debridement is required in cases of osteomyelitis or when the wound involves a deep abscess or spreading tissue infection. Sharp debridement, which can be performed at the bedside, is an option when surgery isn't necessary or the patient is a poor surgical candidate. (For important information on wound debridement, see Chapter 3, page 74.)

Biotherapies

Growth factors and living skin equivalents are two forms of biotherapy that may be included in the care plan for a patient with a diabetic foot ulcer.

Growth factors

Growth factors orchestrate healing in the wound bed. One factor in particular – platelet-derived growth factor (PDGF) – is called the master factor. PDGF plays a central role by stimulating chemotaxis and the proliferation of neutrophils, fibroblasts and monocytes. However, this therapy also relies on an adequate vascular supply, proper wound bed preparation and glycaemic control.

Living skin equivalents

Living skin equivalents are products composed of living cells and a matrix, or scaffolding, that serves as the extracellular medium. These products act as interactive wound coverings, providing growth factors and other needed molecules. Dermagraft® is one example of a living skin equivalent. It has viable fibroblasts that may enhance wound healing rates in diabetic ulcers (Robertshaw 1998).

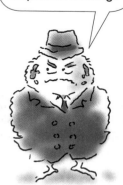

Foiled again! Using a topical antimicrobial on the wound bed helps keep out microorganisms like me. That improves healing!

Living skin equivalents, such as Dermagraft and Apligraf, contribute viable fibroblasts that enhance diabetic ulcer healing.

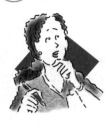

Quick quiz

1. The single greatest risk factor for diabetic foot ulcers is:
   A. PVD
   B. peripheral neuropathy
   C. retinitis pigmentosa
   D. myopathy.

Answer: B. Peripheral neuropathy is the primary risk factor for diabetic foot ulcers.

2. Diabetic ulceration can commonly be found:
   A. around the ankle
   B. over the sacrum
   C. on the dorsal surface of the foot
   D. on the plantar surface of the foot.

Answer: D. Always check the plantar surfaces of the feet for signs of ulcerations. Also check between toes and on the tips of toes.

3. Which complication commonly results from motor neuropathy?
   A. Charcot's neuropathic osteoarthropathy
   B. diminished sensation
   C. clawed toes
   D. poor circulation.

Answer: C. Clawed toes commonly result from motor neuropathy, a long-term complication of diabetes.

4. What may the presence of bone in the wound bed indicate?
   A. neuropathic ulcer
   B. osteomyelitis
   C. loss of sensation
   D. fungal infection.

Answer: B. Bone may be palpated in the wound bed of a patient with osteomyelitis.

5. The 10 g monofilament test is used to assess:
   A. blood flow to the feet
   B. protective sensation of the feet
   C. pressure on the feet
   D. temperature of the feet.

Answer: B. During the 10 g monofilament test, the assessor uses a monofilament to assess the patient's protective sensation, or the ability to detect stimuli that may be harmful to the feet.

6. Which statement about the total contact cast is true?
   A. It's a method of relieving pressure on the foot.
   B. It's a special cast for fractures due to Charcot's neuropathic osteoarthropathy.
   C. It's recommended for use over infected diabetic foot ulcerations.
   D. It's removable.

Answer: A. The total contact cast is an off-loading device that relieves pressure on the foot. However, because it isn't removable, it isn't recommended for use over infected wounds.

Scoring

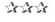 If you answered all six questions correctly, you've got a reason to grin! You off-loaded this quiz in a jiffy.

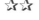 If you answered five questions correctly, brag to your friends! You zipped through this quiz with no pressure.

 If you answered fewer than five questions correctly, don't worry! Put your best foot forward and try again.

References

Cooper, R. (2004) A review of the evidence for the use of topical antimicrobial agents in wound care. *World Wide Wounds.* [on-line] [Accessed on 13/08/08] Available: http://www.worldwidewounds.com/2004/february/Cooper/Topical-Antimicrobial-Agents.html

Department of Health (2007) *About Diabetes.* [online] [Accessed on 24/07/08] Available: http://www.dh.gov.uk/en/Healthcare/NationalServiceFrameworks/Diabetes/DH_074762

Diabetes.co.uk (2008) *Diabietes and Amputation.* [online] [Accessed 24/07/08] Available: http://www.diabetes.co.uk/diabetes-and-amputation.html

Edmonds, M. (2007) Diabetic foot ulcers. In *Skin Breakdown: The Silent Epidemic.* Hull: Smith and Nephew Foundation.

Lavery, L.A., Armstrong, D.G. and Harkless L.B. (1997) Classification of diabetic foot wounds: the University of Texas San Antonio diabetic wound classification system. *Ostomy/Wound Management* 43(2):44–53.

National Institute of Health and Clinical Excellence (2007a) *Scope: Type 1 Diabetes: Diagnosis and Management of Type 1 Diabetes in Primary and Secondary Care.* [on-line] [Accessed on 13/08/08] Available: http://www.nice.org.uk/guidance/index.jsp?action=byID&o=10944

National Institute of Health and Clinical Excellence (2007b) *Specifying A Foot Care Service for People with Diabetes*. [on-line] [Accessed on 13/08/08] Available: http://www.nice.org.uk/

National Institute of Health and Clinical Excellence (NICE) (2008) *CG66 – Diabetes type 2 (update): Full Guideline*.[online] [Accessed on 24/07/08] Available: http://www.nice.org.uk/Guidance/CG66/Guidance/pdf/English

Pecoraro, R.E., Reiber, G.E. and Burgess, E.M. (1990) Pathways to diabetic limb amputation. Basis for prevention. *Diabetes Care* 13(5): 513–521.

Reiber, G.E. (2001) Epidemiology of foot ulcers and amputations in the diabetic foot. In Bowker, J.H. and Pfeifer, M.A. (eds). *Levin and O'Neal's The Diabetic Foot*. 6th edn. St. Louis: Mosby.

Robbins, C.M. (2007) Tinea Pedis. *eMedicine*. [on-line] [Accessed on 13/08/08] Available at http://www.emedicine.com/derm/topic470.htm

Robertshaw, D.A. (1998) The use of Dermagraft in diabetic foot ulceration. *Practical Diabetes International*. 16(4):119–121.

Wagner, F.W. (1981) The dysvascular foot: a system for diagnosis and treatment. *Foot and Ankle* 2(2):64–122.

10 Leg ulcers

Just the facts

In this chapter, you'll learn:

♦ characteristics of venous, arterial and lymphatic ulcers
♦ causes of leg ulcers
♦ assessment criteria for leg ulcers
♦ methods for diagnosing the ulcer type
♦ treatment options for leg ulcers.

A look at leg ulcers

The vascular system is composed of arteries, veins, capillaries and lymphatics. Pressure from the beating heart carries blood away from the heart through the arteries into progressively smaller vessels until they connect with the capillaries. On the other side of the capillaries, small veins receive blood and pass it into progressively larger veins on its return trip to the heart. The lymphatic system is a separate system of vessels that collect waste products and deliver them to the venous system.

Leg ulcers are chronic wounds that most often stem from disorders in the venous, arterial and lymphatic systems. Venous and arterial ulcers are most common in the lower leg while lymphatic ulcers could also occur in the arms or the legs. Venous ulcers account for 70% to 90% of all leg ulcers (Briggs and Closs 2003).

The underlying cause of the ulcer may also be due to a mix of venous and arterial disease (approximately 20%) and a small percentage of ulcers (approximately 5%) can have other causes such as malignancy. Other causes may be vasculitic conditions such as rheumatoid arthritis, blood disorders such as sickle cell disease, diseases such as pyoderma gangrenosum or even practitioner induced wounds (iatrogenic), for example, by applying bandages too tightly (Morison and Moffatt 2007).

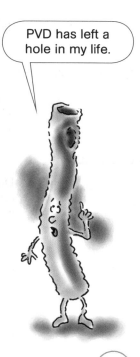

PVD has left a hole in my life.

Venous ulcers

Venous ulcers, which result from venous hypertension, occur on the lower leg. They affect about 1% of the population as a whole but are most common in older adults, affecting approximately 3.5% of the population older than age 65.

Venous anatomy and function

In the circulatory system, arteries carry blood away from the heart, and veins carry blood back to the heart. Capillaries connect these two systems. On the venous side, venules are the small veins that receive blood from the capillaries and deliver it to the larger veins for its return trip to the heart.

Types of veins

In the lower portion of the body, where venous ulcers develop, there are three major types of veins: superficial veins, perforator veins and deep veins.

Skin deep

Superficial veins (e.g. long or short saphenous veins) lie just beneath the skin and drain into deep veins through perforator veins. Varicose veins are superficial veins that have become stretched and tortuous.

Central connectors

Perforator veins connect the superficial veins to the deep veins. Their name is derived from the fact that they perforate the deep fasciae as they connect superficial veins to the deep venous system.

U-turns

Deep veins receive venous blood from the perforator veins and return it to the heart. The major deep veins in the leg include the posterior tibial veins, anterior tibial veins, peroneal veins and the popliteal veins. Each of these veins parallels a corresponding artery. (See *Major lower limb veins*, page 225.)

Vein walls and valves

Compared to arteries of the same size, veins have thinner walls and wider diameters. Vein walls have three distinct layers: an inner, endothelial layer (tunica intima); a middle layer of smooth muscle (tunica media); and an outer, supportive layer (tunica adventitia).

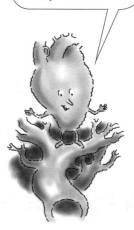

Miles of arteries, arterioles, capillaries, venules and veins keep blood circulating from the heart to every functioning cell in the body – and back.

Major lower limb veins

Venous ulcers most commonly occur in the lower extremities. This illustration shows the major veins in this part of the body.

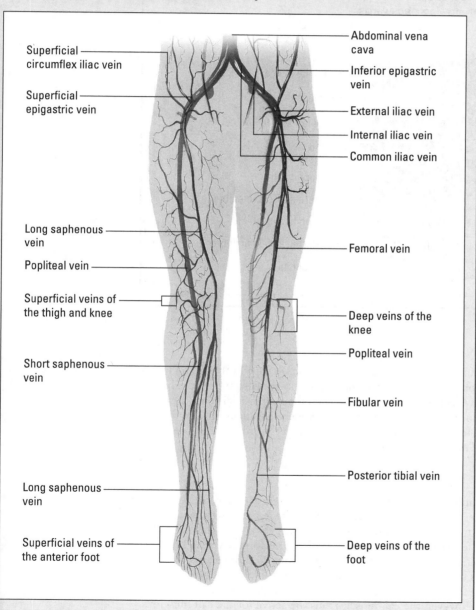

Superficial circumflex iliac vein

Superficial epigastric vein

Long saphenous vein

Popliteal vein

Superficial veins of the thigh and knee

Short saphenous vein

Long saphenous vein

Superficial veins of the anterior foot

Abdominal vena cava

Inferior epigastric vein

External iliac vein

Internal iliac vein

Common iliac vein

Femoral vein

Deep veins of the knee

Popliteal vein

Fibular vein

Posterior tibial vein

Deep veins of the foot

A close look at a vein

This cross-section of a vein clearly illustrates the three layers of the vein wall and its unique cup-shaped valves. These valves open towards the heart and, when closed, prevent blood from flowing backwards.

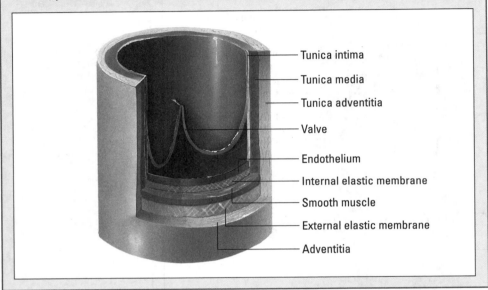

- Tunica intima
- Tunica media
- Tunica adventitia
- Valve
- Endothelium
- Internal elastic membrane
- Smooth muscle
- External elastic membrane
- Adventitia

Veins also have a unique system of cup-shaped valves. The valves function to keep blood flowing in one direction – towards the heart. Deep veins have more of these valves than superficial veins, and veins in the lower leg have more of these valves than veins in the thigh. In perforator veins, the valves open towards the deep veins. (See *A close look at a vein*.)

Pump it up!

Calf muscles have an important role in venous circulation. As calf muscles contract, they squeeze veins in the leg, forcing venous blood towards the heart. When they relax, veins in the leg expand and refill with blood from superficial and perforator veins. This pumping action is important because about 90% of venous blood travels to the heart this way. The other 10% of venous blood empties directly into the vena cava from the great saphenous vein. However, the calf muscles must be active for the calf muscle pump to work. Activity such as walking, ankle flexing and rotation exercises and repeated moving from feet on floor to standing on tiptoes all activate the calf muscle pump. Leg muscle paralysis or prolonged inactivity eliminates the calf muscle pump and inhibits venous blood flow.

Causes

Venous ulcers are due to venous hypertension, which results from venous insufficiency (impaired flow of venous blood from the legs to the heart). In most cases, incompetent valves are to blame. Valve incompetency may be caused by a thrombus (blood clot) that renders the valve useless or by venous wall distention that separates valve cusps to the point where they no longer meet when the valve closes. Trauma and surgery involving leg veins, as well as pregnancy, can affect the veins in the lower leg.

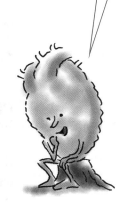

I think I get it! Venous insufficiency causes venous hypertension, which can cause venous ulcers.

The pressure's rising

When the flow of venous blood slows, blood pools in the veins of the lower limbs and venous pressure rises. As the disease progresses, blood backs up through the perforator veins into superficial veins, causing varicose veins to develop in the superficial system. In many cases, oedema develops as excess interstitial fluid accumulates in the tissue of the lower leg. Keep in mind, however, that a patient with varicose veins may not have deep vein insufficiency; vascular tests can differentiate between these two problems.

Venous ulcers can occur in patients with superficial or perforator disease as well as those with deep vein disease. In all cases, the underlying problem is usually venous hypertension.

Warning signs

Initially, venous ulcer development doesn't produce symptoms. The patient may report a general discomfort or aching in the affected areas. Oedema may increase and the skin may feel itchy.

Assessment

Proper assessment of venous ulcers includes collecting a thorough history and performing a physical examination.

History

Develop a complete history of the patient's experience with venous ulcers. Obtain answers to such questions as:

- When did the patient first notice the ulcer?
- Is this the first time that the patient has had an ulcer or is this a recurrence?
- If it's a recurrence, what type of treatment did the patient receive in the past?
- What type of pain management proved effective?
- Does the patient have a history of varicose veins? Venous thromboses? Arterial disease? Bleeding problems of any type? Leg trauma? Leg swelling? Leg surgery?
- Does the patient use tobacco?
- Is there a family history of varicose veins and/or leg ulcers.

Physical examination

Record the size of the ulcer (length, width and depth) and its location. Note any necrosis, exudate (wound fluid) or oedema. Record the patient's description of pain associated with the ulcer. Pain may vary from non-existent to extreme pain and pain levels are often underestimated by practitioners. Sometimes venous ulcer pain is related to oedema around the ankle and the pain reduces when the leg is elevated and the oedema reduces. Pain associated with arterial disease would worsen with leg elevation as the oxygenated blood supply would be reduced (Vowden and Vowden 2007).

Venous ulcers may occur anywhere from the ankle to mid-calf; however, they're most common on the medial aspect of the ankle above the malleolus and may extend all the way around the leg. Most have an irregular shape and are reasonably superficial in depth. The borders may have dry crusts or may be moist and slightly macerated from exudate. The ulcer itself is shallow with a base of red granulation tissue. The surface may be covered by a yellow film (slough) or grey /black necrotic tissue.

Check for oedema and other signs of venous insufficiency. (See *Signs of venous insufficiency*, page 229.) Ask the patient if the oedema gets worse during the day, especially if they have been standing or sitting for long periods. Look at the shape of the leg, is the shape normal; the ankle of a smaller circumference than the calf, is there some bulk to the calf muscle? If the leg is the same circumference up to the knee the patient is likely to have poor calf muscle action. Is there movement in the ankle; a fixed ankle joint may mean the calf muscle is unable to flex as normal.

Are there any varicose veins visible? Look for small broken veins on the inner aspect of the ankle as these indicate venous hypertension affecting tiny superficial blood vessels.

Signs of venous insufficiency

In a patient with venous insufficiency, check for ulcerations around the ankle. Pulses are present but may be difficult to find if oedema is present. Oedema may increase if the foot is dependent for long periods.

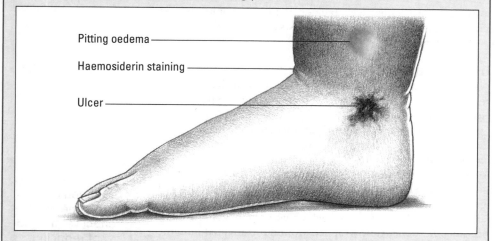

Pitting oedema

Haemosiderin staining

Ulcer

Colouring in

Look at the skin. Does it appear normal or is there dry flaky skin, or even signs of eczema; these can be indicative of venous insufficiency. In venous insufficiency, red blood cells (RBCs), fluid and fibrin leak into tissues. Note the colour of the patient's skin. Hyperpigmentation (haemosiderin staining) is common even when ulcers aren't present. This colour change is due to a buildup of hemosiderin in the interstitial tissue as the RBCs that have leaked into the tissue break down. The fibrin causes skin and subcutaneous tissue to thicken and become fibrotic – a condition called *lipodermatosclerosis*.

On the look out

Other skin changes characteristic of venous insufficiency include oedema, eczema and atrophie blanche:
• Odema is one of the first signs of venous disease. It may be confined to the foot or the ankle or may involve the entire leg.
• Eczema is common, especially in patients who have recurrent ulcers. Skin over scar tissue and oedematous tissue is fragile. Exudate drainage from larger ulcers – or medications themselves – can irritate the skin and aggravate eczema.

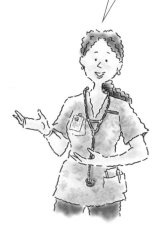

Watch for skin changes that are characteristic of venous insufficiency, including hyperpigmentation, oedema, eczema and atrophie blanche.

- Atrophie blanche may appear as spots of ivory – white plaque in the skin, usually surrounded by hyperpigmentation. Some patients feel discomfort or extreme pain in these areas.

Diagnostic tests

Diagnostic tests for venous ulcers include plethysmography, venous duplex scanning and venography. These tests are generally carried out in vascular laboratories.

Plethysmography

Plethysmography records changes in the volumes and sizes of extremities by measuring changes in blood volume. Types of plethysmography include:
- air plethysmography – which uses an inflatable pneumatic cuff placed around the limb to obtain volume measurements and standing and walking pressures
- photoplethysmography – which uses infrared light transmitted through the skin to measure venous reflux and filling times; delayed healing can be predicted by abnormal filling times
- strain-gauge plethysmography – which uses a mercury-filled, fine bore silicone rubber tube wrapped around the affected limb to measure blood flow and vascular resistance
- impedance plethysmography – which measures the change in resistive impedance of an electrical current as it passes through a body segment.

Venous duplex scanning

Venous duplex scanning is used to assess venous patency and reflux by measuring and recording venous pressures along an extremity as its veins are compressed and released. An experienced technician can use venous duplex scanning to identify thrombosis within a vein and determine whether it's acute or chronic as well as assess venous reflux and the status of valve function. The accuracy of the results may depend on the technician's skill.

Venography

Venography is the radiographic examination of a vein that has been injected with a contrast medium. In the past, this was the only test available to evaluate venous thrombosis; however, with the advent of newer non-invasive tests, venography is rarely used today.

Treatment

Effective treatment of a venous ulcer involves caring for the wound and managing the underlying venous disease. Controlling oedema is the most important goal in managing chronic venous

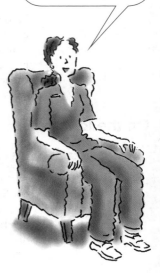

I need a leg up! The most effective method of reducing oedema in a patient with venous ulcers is to raise the affected extremity higher than the heart.

insufficiency. Methods to control oedema include elevation of the affected limb, compression therapy and, sometimes, medication or surgery. Compression therapy is the most important part of the treatment.

Elevation of the limb

An effective method of reducing oedema is to elevate the leg and allow gravity to drain fluid from it. This is best accomplished with the patient in bed with their legs elevated above the level of their heart, or at least higher than the hips. However, a patient with a cardiac or pulmonary condition may find this position intolerable. In this case, any elevation that the patient can tolerate is beneficial. Exercise is very important too, walking is best but any movement that flexes the calf muscle is good.

Compression therapy

Compression therapy is the most effective way of managing oedema, reducing venous hypertension and allowing venous ulcers to heal. However, before applying compression therapy to the patient's treatment regimen, assess their ABPI to ensure the adequacy of arterial blood supply. (See Chapter 9, *Ankle–brachial index*, page 231.) Compression therapy is applied in a specific way to ensure that there is graduated compression up the leg with a higher pressure at the ankle than at the knee. The pressures involved are generally up to 40 mmHg at the ankle so it is vital that the patient is properly assessed and that the person applying the bandage is fully trained and accountable for the procedure. Otherwise that patient could be at significant risk of serious injury.

In stiff pursuit

Calf muscle contractions are key to the effectiveness of compression therapy. As the patient walks or otherwise flexes the calf muscle the compression restricts outwards movement of the calf muscle, directing more of the contraction force inwards and improving the function of the calf muscle pump and, in turn, venous circulation. Therefore, compression therapy has less effect for a sedentary or bedridden patient, which means that any encouragement to flex the calf muscle is very important.

Compression bandages

There are a variety of ways to apply compression therapy. The most common for active ulcers is bandaging. This comes in a variety of forms, mainly elastic or inelastic materials and in multiple layers depending on the bandage type. Bandages are generally worn for up to a week at a time.

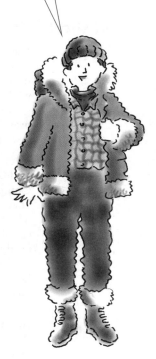

Sometimes layers are a must. Layered compression bandages protect the skin, absorb moisture and provide compression.

Elastic bandages

Elastic bandages for compression may be long stretch or short stretch.

The long . . .

Elastic bandages are long-stretch bandages so called because they can stretch to more than 140% of their length. Long-stretch bandages maintain a constant pressure which rises when the calf muscle is flexed.

. . . and short of it

A short-stretch or inelastic bandage has limited elastic stretch, typically less than 90% of its length. When stretched to its limit, a short-stretch bandage becomes semirigid, providing compression while the patient is active. When the patient rests, the bandage provides less compression, protecting their skin from unnecessary pressure. This type of bandage provides high-working pressure and low-resting pressure.

Multi-layer compression bandages

Compression therapy is applied to the leg from the toes to the knee using 3 or 4 layers. The first layer is soft wool padding which protects the skin and absorbs moisture. It is applied in a spiral with a 50% overlap in each turn. This layer can also be used to fill in concave areas such as behind the ankle to ensure a uniform pressure from the bandages. The padding layer can also be used to help shape the leg so that the calf circumference is more than the ankle to ensure a graduated shape. The next layer is a crepe bandage used to smooth the padding ready for the compression layers. The third layer is a light compression bandage that provides about 17 mmHg of pressure when it is applied in a figure of 8 pattern with a 50% overlap. The final layer is a cohesive (sticks to itself not the patient) compression bandage that provides 23 mmHg of pressure when applied in a spiral with a 50% overlap.

Sometimes it is desirable to have less pressure applied and layer 3 or 4 may be omitted. This may be due to pain or if there is some reduction in the arterial blood flow to the leg (see ABPI).

Two-layer elastic systems

There are some bandage systems which have a foam or padding first layer and a single elastic compression bandage on top.

Compression hosiery

Compression hosiery (socks or stockings) also apply graduated compression therapy to the leg. They can be used to heal the ulcer but are more commonly used to help manage the venous disease and reduce the risk of the ulcer recurring after healing. They are available in 4 classes although class 1–3 are the most commonly used. The higher the class the more pressure, and the more effective they are but they also become increasingly difficult to put on, especially if the patient or their carer has problems such as arthritis, back problems or obesity.

Hosiery comes in full length or knee length and the choice is up to the person who is to wear them. Some people with very large legs where it is difficult to see the knee are likely to need full length.

Intermittent compression therapy (IPC)

Compression pumps may be used in conjunction with support stockings or bandages. These devices are available with sleeves that intermittently inflate. They may have a single chamber or separate bladders that inflate sequentially. The patient may have this therapy for 30 minutes to an hour at a time, at least once a week.

Medication

Medications are rarely prescribed to treat venous ulcers. Antibiotics may be ordered to treat infection. Diuretics shouldn't be prescribed to treat oedema in cases of venous insufficiency because oedema is typically treated in these cases with compression, exercise and limb elevation. If the patient has concomitant heart failure, diuretics may be prescribed to treat it. Because diuretics can cause volume depletion and serious metabolic disorders, monitor the patient closely.

> If diuretics are prescribed to treat a patient with concomitant heart failure, monitor the patient carefully for volume depletion and metabolic disorders.

Surgery

Venous ulcers are a chronic disorder that heal slowly and recur frequently (Bentley 2001). The recurrence rate when no compression is worn could be 60% or higher, and even when compression hosiery is used could still be about 28% (Moffatt and Dorman 1995). Consequently, surgery is rarely a viable treatment. Large surface defects may require repair by skin grafting; however, this is a temporary solution. The underlying problem of venous hypertension remains and, in time, oedema beneath the scar tissue breaks down the scar and creates another ulcer in the same area or nearby. A surgical procedure called subfascial endoscopic perforator surgery (SEPS) may be performed. During this procedure, faulty perforator veins are located and ligated, redirecting blood flow to healthy veins and improving ulcer healing. A more popular recent procedure for varicose vein treatment is foam sclerotherapy where foam is injected into the vein causing the lining to break down and be absorbed by surrounding tissue (NICE, 2007).

Wound care

In general, the simpler the dressing the better. Patients with venous disease can have very sensitive and fragile legs, therefore the dressing should be low adherent, perhaps coated with silicone or other material to reduce the risk of sticking. Other, more interactive, dressings may be used if there is a need to moisten a dry wound, absorb excess exudate or reduce wound pain. (See Chapter 4, *Wound dressings*, page 82.)

And introducing . . .

Newer therapies can also aid in healing chronic venous ulcers. Preliminary studies show that growth factors or protease inhibitors could be used to improve the healing rates in venous ulcers but the treatment can be costly and it is not yet possible to ascertain what the specific problem is at cell level (Krishnamoorthy *et al.* 2001). (For more information on adjunctive therapies, see Chapter 10, *Therapeutic modalities*.)

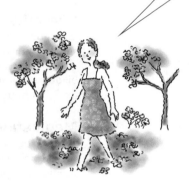

Be sure to choose the proper dressing for your patient with a venous ulcer. Now, if only choosing the right dress was that easy!

Arterial ulcers

Arterial ulcers, which are also called ischaemic ulcers, are the result of tissue ischaemia due to arterial insufficiency. They can occur at the distal (farthest) end of any arterial branch. Arterial ulcers account for 5% to 20% of all leg ulcers (Moffatt *et al.* 2007).

Arterial anatomy and function

Like vein walls, artery walls have three layers:
• tunica intima (innermost layer) – composed of a single layer of endothelial cells on a layer of connective tissue
• tunica media (middle layer) – composed of a thick layer of smooth-muscle cells, collagen and elastic fibres
• tunica adventitia (strong outer layer) – composed of connective tissue, collagen and elastic fibres. (See *A close look at an artery*, page 235.)

With every beat of my heart

Arteries carry blood leaving the heart to every functioning cell in the body. Their strong, muscular walls allow expansion and relaxation

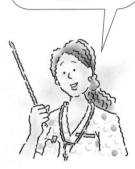

Arterial ulcers account for 5% to 20% of all leg ulcers.

A close look at an artery

This cross-section of an artery illustrates the layers that comprise the arterial wall.

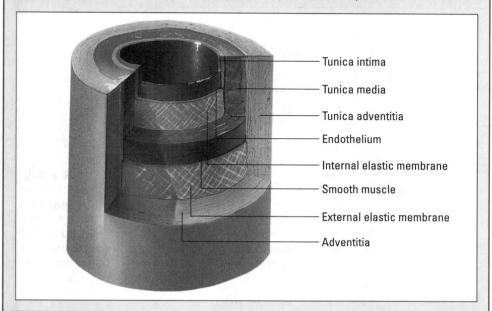

- Tunica intima
- Tunica media
- Tunica adventitia
- Endothelium
- Internal elastic membrane
- Smooth muscle
- External elastic membrane
- Adventitia

with each heartbeat, smoothing the powerful pulse to an almost constant pressure by the time blood reaches the capillaries. The lower portion of the body receives its arterial flow through the abdominal aorta and the major arteries that branch from it. (See *Major lower limb arteries*, page 236.)

Causes

Arterial insufficiency occurs when arterial blood flow is interrupted by an obstruction or arterial stenosis (narrowing of an artery). Occlusion can occur in any artery – from the aorta to a capillary – and can result from trauma or chronic ailment.

The origins of occlusion

The most common cause of occlusion is atherosclerosis. Patients at highest risk for atherosclerosis include men, cigarette smokers and individuals with diabetes mellitus, hyperlipidemia or hypertension. Advanced age places patients at even greater risk. (See *Ageing and arterial insufficiency*.)

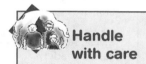

Handle with care

Ageing and arterial insufficiency

When assessing elderly patients, be alert for signs of arterial insufficiency. As ageing occurs, the tunica intima thickens and loses elasticity. Thickening of the intima is one cause of arterial stenosis, which puts older adults at greater risk for arterial insufficiency.

Major lower limb arteries

This illustration identifies the major arteries in the lower portion of the body.

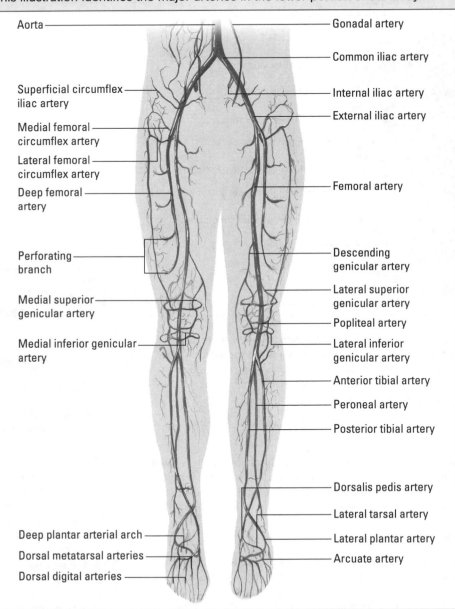

Aorta

Superficial circumflex iliac artery

Medial femoral circumflex artery

Lateral femoral circumflex artery

Deep femoral artery

Perforating branch

Medial superior genicular artery

Medial inferior genicular artery

Gonadal artery

Common iliac artery

Internal iliac artery

External iliac artery

Femoral artery

Descending genicular artery

Lateral superior genicular artery

Popliteal artery

Lateral inferior genicular artery

Anterior tibial artery

Peroneal artery

Posterior tibial artery

Dorsalis pedis artery

Lateral tarsal artery

Lateral plantar artery

Arcuate artery

Deep plantar arterial arch

Dorsal metatarsal arteries

Dorsal digital arteries

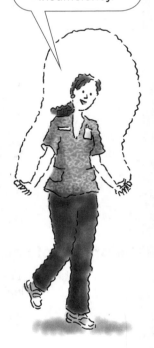

Claudication pain in the calf, thigh or buttocks that's brought on by exercise and is relieved by rest may be the first sign of arterial insufficiency.

Warning signs

In many cases, no signs of arterial insufficiency are apparent until the affected individual suffers an injury. As the demand for additional blood flow to the site of the injury outpaces an occluded artery's ability to deliver blood, ischaemia occurs. Ischaemia is a reduction in the flow of blood to any organ or body part. The primary symptom of ischaemia is pain, which can be severe and may progress from claudication to rest pain.

Claudication

Claudication of the legs is similar to angina of the heart because the cause of both is an insufficient supply of oxygen. In the heart muscle, this oxygen deficiency causes the pain of angina. In leg muscles, the same deficiency causes the pain of claudication.

Claudication, which can occur in any muscle distal to a narrowed artery, is brought on by exercise and is relieved by rest. Typically, patients report claudication pain in the calf, thigh or buttocks. It's measured by how far the patient can walk before needing to stop to relieve the pain. Factors that tend to shorten the distance travelled before pain occurs include obesity, smoking and progressive atherosclerotic disease.

Claudication occurs at a specific distance and is reproducible. Patients experiencing claudication don't have to sit or adopt a particular position to relieve the discomfort; merely stopping reduces the oxygen demand and relieves the pain. As arterial insufficiency progresses, the distance shortens until, ultimately, the patient feels pain even when resting.

Rest pain

Rest pain commonly occurs in the foot and can occur when the patient is asleep. Getting up and walking may provide some relief; however, walking isn't the key – lowering the extremity is. Gravity helps blood flow into the foot and calf, reducing the oxygen deficit and relieving discomfort. By the time rest pain occurs, tissues in the foot are severely ischaemic, whether or not an ulcer is present. This means that the foot is very vulnerable to trauma and needs to be protected. Pain needs to be carefully assessed and treated; the use of opiate analgesia may be necessary. Unless arterial flow is restored, the patient may need amputation.

Rest pain in the foot is more likely to be reduced by lowering the foot than by walking. Gravity helps blood flow into the foot, reducing the oxygen deficit and relieving discomfort.

Assessment

Assessment of arterial ulcers requires collecting a thorough patient history and performing a physical examination.

History

A patient history reveals whether the patient's wound is an arterial ulcer caused by arterial insufficiency. Obtain answers to such questions as:

- Has the patient experienced any pain?
- If he describes intermittent claudication, how far can he walk before pain sets in?
- If the patient says he has pain while resting, when did he first notice it and what measures does he take to relieve the pain?
- If the pain is in his foot, does getting up or hanging that foot over the edge of the bed help relieve the pain?
- What position is most comfortable for the patient? (Many patients spend their nights sleeping in a chair because the arterial pressure in the leg is too low to perfuse tissues while the leg is extended.)

Smoke signals

Ask the patient about smoking as well. If they smoke, determine how long they have been a smoker and how much they smoke.

Physical examination

Start your examination by inspecting the common sites of arterial ulcers: the tips of toes, the corners of nail beds on the toes, over bony prominences and between toes. The edges of arterial ulcers are often well demarcated. Because there's little blood flow to the tissue, the base of the ulcer is pale and dry with little granulation tissue present. You may see an area of wet necrosis or a dry scab. The skin surrounding the ulcer will feel cooler than normal on palpation. (See *Signs of arterial insufficiency*, page 239.)

Next, elevate the foot with the ulcer to a 30-degree angle; the skin colour in an ischaemic foot pales. Then ask the patient to place their foot in a dependent position. Ischaemic skin becomes deep red as the tissue refills with blood. This dramatic colour change is called dependent rubor – a sign of severe tissue ischaemia. The nails may be thin and pale yellow, or they may have thickened due to an existing fungal infection in the nail beds. A Doppler signal may be heard over small arteries, but this doesn't signify blood flow that's sufficient enough to heal the ulcer.

Focus pocus

The specialist will perform a focused examination of the arterial system. The abdominal aorta is palpated to check for the presence of an aortic aneurysm. (In an obese patient, the abdominal aorta won't

Signs of arterial insufficiency

Arterial ulcers most commonly occur in the area around the toes or the top of the foot. In a patient with arterial insufficiency, the foot usually turns deep red when dependent and the nails may be thick and ridged. In addition, pulses may be faint or absent; the skin is cool, pale and shiny; and the patient may report pain in their legs and feet.

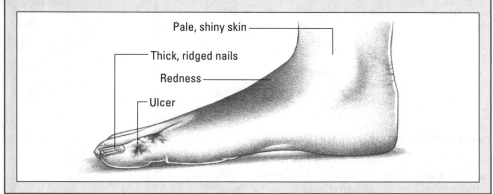

Pale, shiny skin

Thick, ridged nails

Redness

Ulcer

be palpable.) An embolus can occlude an artery and cause ischaemia, and an aortic aneurysm may be the source of the embolus. 'Blue toe syndrome' (a painful, ischaemic toe) is caused by embolic debris in the arteries that supply the toe.

The femoral and popliteal arteries are palpated. You can feel for a pulse over the posterior tibial, anterior tibial, peroneal and dorsalis pedis pulses in each foot. (See *Assessing lower extremity pulses*, page 240.) Keep in mind that an absent dorsalis pedis pulse may not be an abnormal finding. Under normal conditions, some patients don't have a palpable dorsalis pedis pulse. Pulses can be palpated when the pressure is about 70 mmHg. If there's no palpable pulse, the pressure is probably less than 70 mmHg.

Colour chart

Compare the colour of both legs to each other and palpate each leg for temperature. A difference in temperature of 10 degrees or more can be noted by palpation. While the patient lies down, elevate both of their feet about 12 inches (129 cm) or to a 30-degree angle. Watch for a colour change. Compress the great toe bilaterally and compare the capillary refill of each side. Normal tissue should refill in less than 3 seconds.

Assessing lower extremity pulses

These illustrations show where to position your fingers when palpating for pulses of the lower extremities. Use your index and middle fingers to apply pressure.

Posterior tibial pulse

Apply pressure behind and slightly below the medial malleolus.

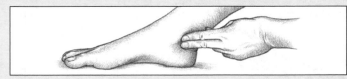

Dorsalis pedis pulse

Place your fingers on the medial dorsum of the foot while the patient points their toes down. The pulse is difficult to palpate here and may seem to be absent in healthy patients.

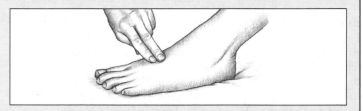

Diagnostic tests

Specialist diagnostic tests commonly used in the vascular laboratory to assess arterial flow to the extremities include segmental pressure recordings, Doppler ultrasonography, duplex ultrasonography, transcutaneous oxygen measurement and arteriography. The ABPI is usually used first in the primary care setting in a specialist leg ulcer clinic or at least by a practitioner qualified in leg ulcer care to obtain an initial idea of the arterial blood supply to the lower leg.

Segmental pressure recordings

Blood pressure is the first test performed to assess the adequacy of arterial blood flow to the legs. Normally, blood pressure readings taken in the arm and the leg should be the same when the patient is

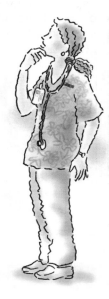

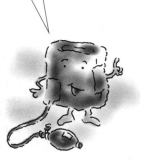

Unequal blood pressure readings in your patient's arms and legs may alert you to problems with the blood flow to their legs.

Vascular ulcers

Vascular ulcers typically result from some form of peripheral vascular disease, which can affect the arterial, venous and lymphatic systems.

Venous ulcers

Venous ulcers are the end stage of venous hypertension, which results from venous insufficiency. The most frequently occurring lower leg ulcers, venous ulcers are typically found in the gaiter region and around the ankle, as shown in the photo below.

Lymphatic ulcers

Lymphatic ulcers result from lymphoedema, in which thickened tissue compresses the capillaries. This occludes blood flow to the skin. These ulcers are extremely difficult to treat because of the reduced blood flow. The photo below shows a patient with lymphoedema of the leg and a large lymphatic ulcer.

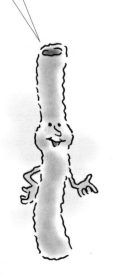

Vascular ulcers differ in appearance and severity, depending on the part of the vascular system that's affected.

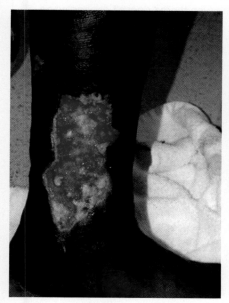

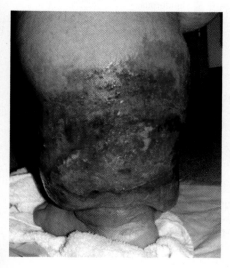

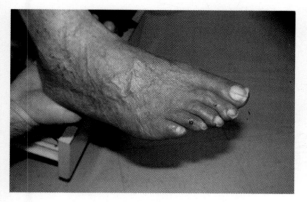

Arterial ulcers

Arterial ulcers result from insufficient blood flow to tissue due to arterial insufficiency. They're commonly found at the distal ends of arterial branches, especially at the tips of the toes, the corners of nail beds or over bony prominences, as shown in the photo on the left.

Categorising pressure ulcers

You can use pressure ulcer characteristics gained from your assessment to categorise a pressure ulcer, as described here. Categorising reflects the anatomic depth of exposed tissue. Keep in mind that if the wound contains necrotic tissue, you won't be able to determine the category until you can see the wound base.

Category I

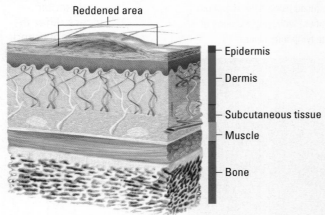

Reddened area

- Epidermis
- Dermis
- Subcutaneous tissue
- Muscle
- Bone

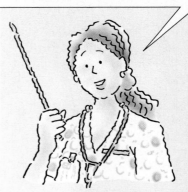

Warning! Category I damage. Non-blanching erythema can be the first sign of tissue destruction but if detected and treated early it may be reversible. Look for discoloration of the skin (may be difficult to detect in darkly pigmented skin), warmth, oedema, hardness and/or pain. Remember, the redness associated with non-blanching erythema doesn't change when compressed.

Now the damage is done but if you start treatment quickly you may prevent further deterioration. Look for partial-thickness skin loss or damage involving both the epidermis and the dermis. Category II presents as a shallow open ulcer without slough or as an intact or ruptured blister.

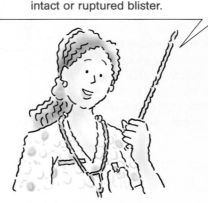

Category II

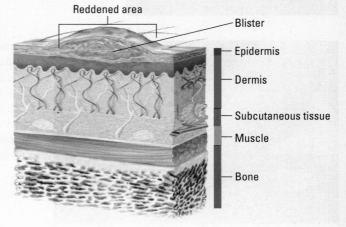

Reddened area

- Blister
- Epidermis
- Dermis
- Subcutaneous tissue
- Muscle
- Bone

Category III

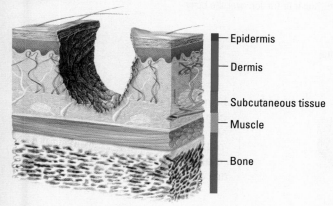

- Epidermis
- Dermis
- Subcutaneous tissue
- Muscle
- Bone

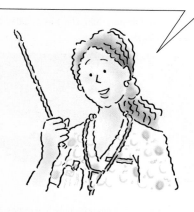

Category III damage is significant and needs urgent attention. These ulcers are full thickness, usually presenting as deep cavities or craters. You may see subcutaneous fat but not bone, tendon or muscle. Some slough may be present and the ulcer may include undermining and tunnelling.

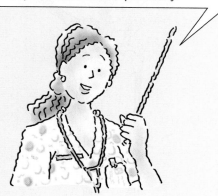

Oh dear, category IV ulcers have full-thickness tissue loss with exposed or palpable bone, tendon or muscle. Slough or eschar may be present as well as undermining and/or tunnelling. Treatment is urgent; category IV ulcers can extend into muscle and other supporting structures making osteomyelitis and osteitis likely to occur. Septicaemia is also a possibility.

Category IV

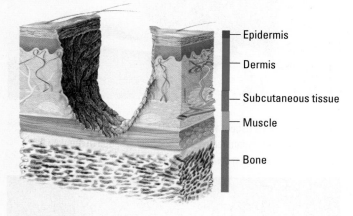

- Epidermis
- Dermis
- Subcutaneous tissue
- Muscle
- Bone

Diabetic foot ulcers

Because of the neurological and vascular complications associated with diabetes, patients with this disorder are prone to foot ulcers. Some develop in response to unrelieved pressure, shear or friction over the bony prominences of the foot, just like pressure ulcers elsewhere on the body.

This photo shows a patient with diabetes who has a pressure wound to the right lateral malleolus. Note the characteristic tissue changes associated with arterial insufficiency: thin, shiny skin; pale colouring; and muscular atrophy in the lower extremity.

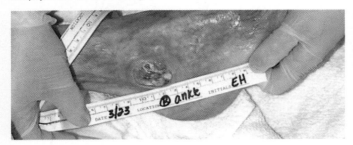

This photo shows a patient with type II diabetes who has developed a pressure ulcer from impaired protective sensation and poor mobility.

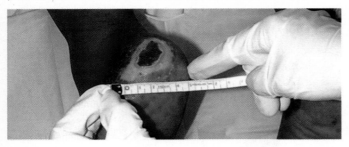

This photo shows a patient who has a diabetic foot ulcer on the plantar surface of the fifth metatarsal head. The circular shape of the wound is consistent with a wound created by pressure over a bony prominence.

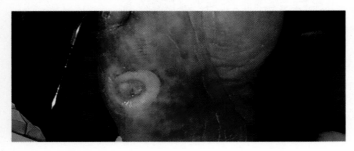

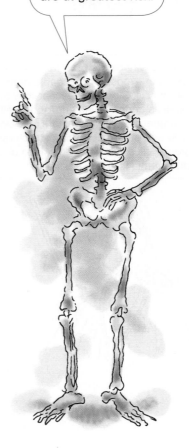

Pressure over bony prominences can cause all sorts of problems. For patients who have diabetes, the feet are at greatest risk.

lying down. A lower reading in the legs indicates an arterial blockage that may be caused by problems, such as a thrombus, cholesterol or pressure on the outside of the artery.

Blood pressure is measured in both arms while the patient is lying down. Then blood pressure is measured at several points along each leg. Each reading is accompanied by a waveform tracing of the pulse. The entire procedure takes only 20 to 30 minutes. In some cases, the procedure is repeated after a short period of controlled exercise. In arterial insufficiency, arterial blood flow during exercise fails to keep up with muscle demand. Changes in the waveforms and Doppler signals should occur at the same time that the patient reports symptoms of claudication.

Doppler ultrasonography

In Doppler ultrasonography, sound waves are used to assess blood flow. This test may be used alone or in conjunction with other diagnostic tests to assess arterial blood flow. During the procedure, a handheld transducer directs high-frequency sound waves into the artery being tested. Sound waves that strike moving RBCs change frequency – a Doppler shift – in relation to the velocity of the RBCs. The practitioner then reviews the graphic record of these waveforms to determine whether an obstruction exists. (See *How the Doppler probe works*.)

How the Doppler probe works

The Doppler ultrasound probe directs high-frequency sound waves through layers of tissue. When the sound waves strike RBCs moving in the bloodstream, the frequency of the sound waves changes in proportion to the velocity of the RBCs. A recording of these waves facilitates detection of arterial and venous obstruction.

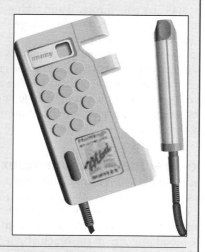

Image reproduced with kind permission of Huntleigh Healthcare, Cardiff.

Duplex ultrasonography

Similar to Doppler ultrasonography, duplex ultrasonography is used to measure blood flow in the arteries and veins of the legs and arms. A transducer probe with conductive gel is placed along different points of the vessel being studied and the data are viewed and recorded on an ultrasound monitor. Duplex ultrasonography can accurately identify areas of thrombosis in the blood vessels.

Transcutaneous oxygen measurement

Some vascular laboratories perform transcutaneous oxygen measurement to assess the perfusion of the microvasculature.

In this test, an electrode is attached to the patient's skin using double-sided tape. Room temperature is kept constant to ensure an accurate reading. Then the patient is monitored for about 20 minutes as the measurement is taken.

A transcutaneous oxygen of about 40 mmHg is generally regarded as the cutoff value associated with inability to heal. However, the accuracy and, in turn, the dependability of this test varies depending on the laboratory and technician.

Arteriography

An invasive procedure that's only performed if the patient agrees to undergo a corrective procedure for any problem discovered, arteriography is performed by inserting a catheter into the arterial system, injecting a radiopaque contrast medium (a contrast medium that X-rays can't pass through) and taking an X-ray as the contrast medium is injected. The resulting image shows the lumen of the artery and any defect present.

The procedure has some disadvantages and significant risks. For example, several medications can't be taken for a time before the procedure. Also, some patients may be allergic to the contrast medium. Possible complications include injury to the artery, which requires emergency surgery, and haematoma, which requires drainage.

Ankle–brachial pressure index

ABPI is a value derived from blood pressure measurements that, taken as a whole, illustrate the progress of arterial disease – or degree of improvement – in the affected limb. Each value or index is a ratio of a blood pressure measurement in the affected limb to the systolic blood pressure in the brachial arteries. Improvement, or lack thereof, becomes clear when the most recent value is compared to prior values.

The index can also be used to assess treatment methods. Comparing a reading taken before surgery, such as bypass surgery or angioplasty, to a reading taken afterwards can indicate the procedure's effectiveness.

Take these steps

When measuring ABPI, you'll use a Doppler ultrasound and a blood pressure cuff.

The steps of the procedure are as follows:
- Place the patient in a horizontal position so the brachial, dorsalis pedis and posterior tibial arteries are at the same level.
- The patient must rest quietly for at least 15–20 minutes to allow time for the blood pressure to equalise and settle.
- Apply ultrasound gel over the brachial pulse site.
- Measure the brachial systolic blood pressure on both arms using the Doppler. If the pressure readings differ, use the higher of the two systolic pressures.
- Wrap the blood pressure cuff around the patient's ankle, just above the malleoli.
- Identify the dorsalis pedis or posterior tibial artery, apply gel to the area and hold the Doppler transducer over the artery at a 45-degree angle.
- Inflate the blood pressure cuff until you can no longer hear the Doppler signal; then slowly deflate the cuff. When the Doppler signal returns, record the pressure. This is the ankle systolic pressure.
- Repeat the procedure for at least one of the other (ideally three) pulses in the foot.
- Calculate the ABPI by dividing the highest ankle pressure reading by the higher of the two brachial systolic pressures. (See *Interpreting ABPI results*.)

> ABPI is calculated by dividing ankle pressure by the higher of two brachial systolic pressures.

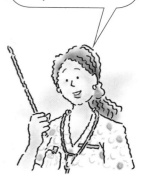

Interpreting ABPI results

This chart will help you interpret ABPI calculations. Keep in mind that ABPI results aren't reliable for patients with diabetes.

ABPI	Interpretation
> 0.8 to 1.3	Normal
0.5 to 0.8	Claudication
0.2 to 0.5	Resting ischaemic pain
< 0.2	Gangrene

Treatment

The first goal in the treatment of an arterial ulcer is re-establishing arterial flow. Without oxygenated blood, the ulcer won't heal. Options for revascularisation include angioplasty and stents or less commonly arterial bypass surgery. In addition, the ulcer must receive appropriate wound care. In general, medications aren't effective when arterial insufficiency has advanced to the point that ulcers are present.

Arterial bypass surgery

Arterial bypass is the gold standard for restoring arterial flow. The type and extent of bypass surgery depends on the ulcer's stage and location and the patient's general health. The graft may be autogenous (a vessel taken from the patient) or a synthetic material, typically Dacron or polytetrafluoroethylene.

Angioplasty and stents

Less invasive interventions, such as angioplasty, are more commonly used for treatment of arterial stenosis. During angioplasty, a catheter with a balloon is inserted into the patient's artery. Using fluoroscopy, the surgeon carefully manoeuvres the catheter to the portion of the artery narrowed by plaque and then expands the balloon. The expanding balloon crushes the plaque against the wall of the artery, increasing the lumen diameter.

Stents are small metal structures that can be inserted into an artery after angioplasty to hold the artery open. They were developed to extend the amount of time that the artery remains open after angioplasty and reduce the need for surgery. Stent placement is gaining in popularity but the success rate of this procedure over time has yet to be determined. However, stents may be an alternative for a patient who's considered too high risk for surgery.

Wound care

In general, keep arterial ulcers dry and protected from pressure. Avoid soaking arterial ulcers. Ischaemic tissue macerates in water, increasing the extent of tissue loss and promoting bacterial proliferation. Care must be taken with adhesive dressings and tapes as the skin is very vulnerable to trauma, their use should be avoided.

Foot care

Make sure the patient's foot is protected at all times. Consider using a large bulky dressing or protective footgear – there are many types

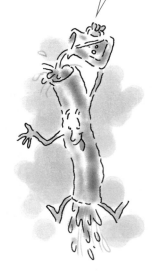

The first treatment goal for arterial ulcers is to re-establish arterial flow. This can be achieved through bypass surgery or angioplasty and stents.

to choose from. If the patient is mobile ensure they can walk safely. Keep in mind that ischaemic tissue can easily develop additional ulcers with little irritation or pressure. Even pressure from the foot resting on the bed or an ill-fitting protective boot can initiate new ulcers. If your patient opts for foot protection, check the device carefully for possible pressure points.

If the ulcer area is a digit and contains necrotic tissue or develops dry gangrene, continue to apply a dry dressing. Reassure the patient that a necrotic digit won't cause further harm. However, these areas have no sensation and must be protected from injury. If loss of a toe seems imminent, explain this to the patient and let them talk about their feelings. Having a necrotic toe fall off is a shocking and frightening event for most patients, but it's even more devastating when the patient isn't prepared for it.

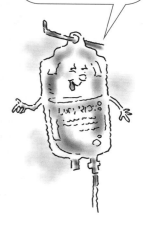

Ischaemic tissue that becomes infected may need to be treated with I.V. antibiotics. That's why I'm hanging around.

Toe the line

Carefully monitor the line of demarcation between dead and viable tissues. This area is typically painful and easily infected. Treat infected ischaemic tissue with I.V. antibiotics.

If revascularisation succeeds, you'll need to change the type of dressing. At this point, you can treat the wound according to the axiom, 'keep moist tissue moist and dry tissue dry', using any dressing that keeps the wound bed moist and the surrounding tissue dry. The choice of dressing will depend on the treatment objectives and how fragile the skin is. If very fragile then don't use an adhesive dressing. A hydrogel may be used if there is necrotic tissue remaining or if the wound is very dry. A foam, alginate or hydrofibre may be useful if the wound is wet. If you are confident the skin can tolerate it and the wound is not too wet, a hydrocolloid dressing may be helpful.

Lymphatic ulcers

Lymphatic ulcers, which result from injury in the presence of lymphoedema (swelling that results from impaired normal flow of lymph into venous circulation because of obstruction) occur most commonly on the arms and legs. Lymphoedema leaves the skin vulnerable to infection and creates skin folds that trap moisture. These conditions cause ulcerations that become difficult to treat.

Lymphatic anatomy and function

The lymphatic system is a component of the peripheral vascular system. Lymph is a protein-rich fluid similar to plasma. As lymph circulates through lymphatic vessels, it collects wastes, including bacteria, and transports them to lymph nodes. The nodes filter wastes out of the lymph and add lymphocytes to the fluid. Lymph moves slowly through the lymphatic system, driven by muscle contraction and filtration.

Causes

Injury to the swollen tissue caused by lymphoedema may result in an ulcer that's slow to heal.

Lymphoedema may be congenital (primary) or acquired (secondary). Secondary lymphoedema can be caused by surgery that severs or removes lymph nodes – radical mastectomy, for example – or it may result from compression of a vessel or node due to obesity or unrelated chronic swelling. For instance, patients with chronic venous hypertension and insufficiency may eventually develop lymphoedema if venous oedema is poorly managed.

Patients with lymphoedema are prone to skin and soft tissue infections and may require long-term treatment with antibiotics. Prophylactic treatment with antibiotics is common because lymphoedema causes progressive destruction of lymphatic vessels and nodes which, in turn, slowly increases the patient's risk of infection. Recurrent cellulitis (tissue infection) is also commonly seen in patients with lymphoedema.

Hard to handle

In the legs, lymphoedema causes a steady seepage of fluids into interstitial tissue. In time, skin and underlying tissues become firm and fibrotic. Thickened tissue presses on the capillaries and occludes blood flow to the skin. The resulting poor circulation makes the leg ulcers that occur with lymphoedema extremely difficult to treat.

Leg ulcers on lymphoedematous tissue are usually the result of traumatic injury or pressure. However, in extreme cases of lymphoedema, the folds of tissue develop deep fissures that trap moisture, causing tissue maceration and the start of a new ulcer. (See *Lymphatic ulcers and obesity*, page 247.)

Warning signs

The only warning sign of a lymphatic ulcer that a patient may report is a feeling of heaviness. This sensation is caused by oedema in the affected extremity.

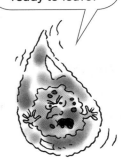

The lymphatic system circulates lymph through vessels to the lymph nodes, where wastes, including bacteria like me, are filtered out. And I didn't even say I was ready to leave!

Handle with care

Lymphatic ulcers and obesity

Disorders such as obesity can induce venous hypertension. The patient who's morbidly obese may already have deep skin folds in which ulceration has developed. Pay close attention to these areas when assessing a bariatric patient for a lymphatic ulcer.

Assessment

Lymphatic ulcers are most common in the ankle area but may develop at any trauma site. Ulcers are shallow and may be oozing, moist or blistered. The surrounding skin is usually firm, fibrotic and thickened by oedema. Cellulitis may be present as well. A diagnosis of lymphoedema is based on the clinical appearance of the skin.

Diagnostic tests

Specific tests for determining whether a patient has a lymphatic ulcer don't exist; however, differentiating a lymphatic disorder from a vascular disorder can be difficult and sometimes they can coexist. Tests should be performed to rule out a vascular problem.

Treatment

Treatment of lymphatic ulcers has two goals: to reduce oedema (and maintain the reduction) and to prevent complications such as infection. Leg elevation is an important part of therapy for patients with lymphoedema. However, in cases of long-standing oedema, elevation may be ineffective. The use of compression pumps and effective wound care are also part of the treatment plan. Skin care is also very important to help prevent further skin breakdown and infection.

Compression pumps

A compression pump is an effective method of reducing oedema. Pump use is a lifelong part of managing oedema. The pump

> The two treatment goals for lymphatic ulcers are reducing oedema and preventing complications such as infection.

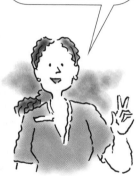

reduces the volume of fluid in a lymphoedematous limb. The pressure should be set low, in the range of 30 to 50 mmHg. After each compression session, the patient must put on compression bandages or another compression garment. Without these, progress gained from the pumping is lost as soon as the patient stands or sits upright.

In addition, comprehensive decongestive therapy is a form of massage that has proven effective for some patients. After each session, the affected limb is wrapped with a short-stretch bandage. This therapy can be combined with compression pump use.

Wound care

Wound care for lymphatic leg ulcers is similar to care for venous ulcers. The primary difference is that the risk of infection is much higher for patients with lymphoedema. In lymphoedema, choose dressings that can manage large fluid loads while protecting surrounding skin, such as foams or other absorbent dressings.

Vascular ulcer care wrap-up

Keep the following tips in mind as you care for a patient with any form of leg ulcer:
* The ulcer is only the tip of the iceberg. It is a sign of an underlying disease. Care must also address the underlying disorder or the ulcer won't heal. For instance, with venous ulcers, the underlying venous hypertension must be treated. With arterial ulcers, arterial blood flow must be restored.
* Vascular disease is pervasive, so look for problems in other areas of the body.
* Be sure to choose the proper dressing for each ulcer. Remember, dressing choice depends on the characteristics of the ulcer as well as the ulcer type and the most important choice to be made is about treating the underlying condition.
* For the most part, the wound care axiom of keeping moist tissue moist and dry tissue dry (i.e. surrounding skin) applies to leg ulcers too. The one exception is an arterial ulcer, which generally should be kept dry until the area is revascularised. Then the axiom applies for arterial ulcers as well.
* Whenever possible, avoid using tape on the patient's skin. Skin affected by vascular disease is fragile and new ulcers form easily.

Patient education

Typically, the success or failure of treatment is in the patient's hands because they have the primary responsibility for caring for this chronic condition. Living with a chronic condition such as venous disease can be difficult for patients and they will need a lot of support. They may be living with pain, discomfort, limitations on their mobility and sore, itchy skin conditions. Patients may react to dressings and lotions; they may find compression bandages and hosiery tight and uncomfortable. All of this should be borne in mind when negotiating care and treatment with the patient. It is not enough to tell a patient what to do. It is important that they are involved in treatment decisions and that an effort is made to help them understand the condition and its management. Be prepared to compromise, empathise and explain, and the person is more likely to engage with you and their care. This approach promotes concordance rather than the outdated compliance model where patients were expected to do as they were told. Concordance is more likely to lead to successful long-term outcomes. Patient teaching should provide clear instructions and rationales to encourage active patient participation.

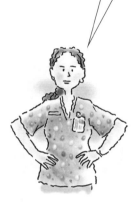

Remember to look for problems in other areas of your patient's body because vascular disease is pervasive.

Tips of the trade

Pass these tips along to the patient to promote leg ulcer healing and reduce the risk of developing new ulcers:
- Look at your skin every day. Use lotion on dry, flaky skin.
- Avoid products with perfumes and additives, they may irritate your skin.
- Use your calf muscles because frequent walks aid healing.
- Flex your feet up and down (as if you were using the pedals in a car) frequently when sitting.
- Elevate your legs whenever you sit.
- Wear shoes that fit well and always wear socks under shoes.
- Wear your compression stockings as directed.
- Don't sit or stand for long periods of time.
- Try to maintain your target weight.
- Report any skin injury to your practitioner.
- Don't smoke.

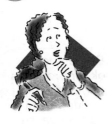

Quick quiz

1. Where's the most common site for a venous ulcer to develop?
A. popliteal area
B. anterior thigh
C. lateral aspect of the foot
D. medial aspect of the ankle.

Answer: D. Venous ulcers are most common on the medial aspect of the ankle above the malleolus and may extend all the way around the leg.

2. Your patient has venous insufficiency. Their leg oedema is best treated by:
A. compression and leg elevation
B. diuretics and compression
C. leg elevation and diuretics
D. restricting fluid intake and compression.

Answer: A. Compression helps to manage oedema when the patient is upright. Leg elevation uses gravity to maximise venous return.

3. ABPI is:
A. a guide to venous hypertension
B. a value that reflects the amount of arterial blood flow to the ankle
C. obtained in a sitting position with feet flat
D. normal if it's above 0.5 mmHg.

Answer: B. In ABPI, each value reflects the ratio of ankle systolic pressure to brachial systolic pressure.

4. The best dressing type for an ischaemic ulcer on the toe is:
A. hydrocolloid
B. wet to dry
C. dry and low adherent
D. hydrogel.

Answer: C. An ischaemic – or arterial – ulcer should be kept dry and protected until blood flow to the area is restored.

5. Which sign or symptom is a key indication of progressive arterial insufficiency?
A. cyanosis when the foot is in a dependent position
B. pain
C. oedema
D. hyperpigmentation of the skin.

Answer: B. Pain is the most common presenting symptom in arterial disease with or without an ulcer.

6. Which therapy is the most effective treatment for managing oedema?

    A.   hydrotherapy

    B.   compression therapy

    C.   ice therapy

    D.   diuretic therapy.

Answer: B. Compression therapy is the most effective way to manage oedema.

7. What test is performed first to assess arterial blood flow to the legs?

    A.   segmental pressure readings

    B.   Doppler ultrasonography

    C.   duplex ultrasonography

    D.   ABPI.

Answer: D. ABPI is usually the first test performed to assess the adequacy of arterial blood flow to the legs.

Scoring

☆☆☆ If you answered all seven questions correctly, take a break! You deserve a splendid evening off tonight.

☆☆ If you answered five or six questions correctly, good for you! You're dancing right through these quizzes.

☆ If you answered fewer than five questions correctly, don't be upset! We're certain that your condition isn't chronic.

References

Bentley, J. (2001) Preventing unnecessary suffering: an audit of a leg ulcer clinic. *British Journal of Community Nursing* 6(3):136–144.

Briggs, M. and Closs, S.J. (2003) The prevalence of leg ulcers: a review of the literature. *EWMA Journal* 3(2):14–20.

Krishnamoorthy, L., Morris, H.L. and Harding, K.G. (2001) Specific growth factors and the healing of chronic wounds. *Journal of Wound Care* 10(5):173–178.

Moffatt, C.J. and Dorman, M.C. (1995) Recurrence of leg ulcers within a community service. *Journal of Wound Care* 4(2):57–61.

Moffatt, C., Martin, R. and Smithdale, R. (2007) Leg ulcer management. In *Arterial Disease*. Chapter 5. pp. 94–123. Oxford: Blackwell.

Morison, M.J. and Moffatt, C.J. (2007) A framework for patient assessment and care planning. In Morison, M.J, Moffatt, C.J. and Franks, P.J. (eds). *Leg Ulcers: A Problem Based Learning Approach*. Chapter 7. London: Mosby.

National Institute of Health and Clinical Excellence (NICE) (2007) Ultrasound guided foam sclerotherapy. Available: http://www.nice.org.uk/Guidance/IPG217/NiceGuidance/pdf/English Accessed on 23th November 2008.

Vowden, P. and Vowden, K. (2007) Ischaemic ulceration: investigation of arterial disease. In Morison, M.J., Moffatt, C.J. and Franks, P.J. (eds). *Leg Ulcers: A Problem Based Learning Approach*. Chapter 16. London: Mosby.

⑪ Accountability and legal issues

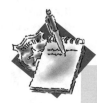

Just the facts

In this chapter, you'll learn:

- ♦ accountability issues
- ♦ standards for healthcare practice
- ♦ patient rights
- ♦ legal issues related to wound care
- ♦ effective record keeping strategies.

A look at accountability

Accountability is about taking responsibility for what you do or do not do. Registered nurses are personally accountable for any actions or omissions in their practice. This means that as a nurse, you must be able to explain (justify) why you cared for a patient in a certain way or took the decisions you did.

All registered nurses in the UK are required to comply with a document called The Code – standards of conduct, performance and ethics for nurses and midwives (NMC 2008a). The Code states that nurses should:

- make the care of people their first concern, treating them as individuals and respecting their dignity
- work with others to protect and promote the health and well-being of those in their care, their families and carers and the wider community
- provide a high standard of practice and care at all times
- be open and honest, act with integrity and uphold the reputation of the nursing profession.

Failure to comply with The Code may raise questions about fitness to practise and possibly endanger the nurse's registration. The Code was produced by the Nursing and Midwifery Council (NMC). The NMC's main purpose is to establish and maintain standards of nurse education, training, conduct and performance in order to safeguard the health and well-being of the general public (NMC 2009).

Nurses are responsible for maintaining the knowledge and skills necessary to practise safely and for ensuring they understand their scope of practice and remain within it. Registered nurses must sign a notification of practice every three years in order to remain on the national nurses register. This register is maintained by the NMC.

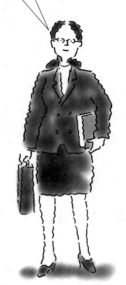

A legal issue is anything questionable in the care you provide that leads to an adverse outcome.

A look at legal issues

Wounds affect thousands of people each year. They contribute to morbidity and mortality, increase the cost of care and, sometimes, contribute to litigation issues. To safeguard your practice, you need to know to what standards you are held in the event of a legal issue. By learning to properly assess, manage and evaluate wounds, you can improve your patients' clinical outcomes. At the same time, you'll minimise the risk of litigation.

What's a legal issue?

A legal issue is anything questionable in provided care that's related to some adverse occurrence or outcome.

Sticking to the issues

Here are some examples of legal issues:
- a possibly negligent action or omission by a healthcare provider
- deviation from an accepted standard of care
- inconsistencies in documentation.

A common question that arises in issues of medical malpractice is, 'Has the clinician met accepted standards of care?' For example, did a nurse fail to implement preventative measures even though a patient was identified as being at risk of pressure ulcers?

Standards of care

Standard of care is a term used to specify what's reasonable under a certain set of circumstances. Standards are used to define certain aspects of a profession, such as:
- the focus of its pursuits
- the beneficiaries of its service
- the responsibilities of its practitioners.

In healthcare, the prevailing professional standard of care is defined as the level of care, skill and treatment deemed acceptable and appropriate by similar healthcare providers. A standard is a yardstick against which effective care can be measured.

Standard issue

Standards for wound care practice are derived from several sources:
- Nursing and Midwifery Council
- Department of Health
- National Institute for Health and Clinical Excellence (NICE)
- Health Care Commission and Health Care Standards Unit
- specialist interest/advisory groups such as the European Pressure Ulcer Advisory Panel (EPUAP) and European Wound Management Association (EWMA)
- local policies and procedures
- job descriptions.

National Institute for Health and Clinical Excellence (NICE)

NICE is an independent organisation responsible for providing evidence-based national guidance on all aspects of healthcare. (See *Spotlight on NICE*.) Guidelines from NICE are a primary source of wound care standards for all healthcare practitioners; subjects to date include Pressure Ulcers, Difficult to Heal Surgical Wounds, Vacuum Assisted Closure, Surgical Site Infection, Nutrition and Eczema.

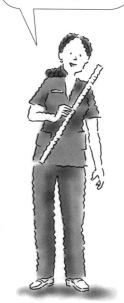

How do you measure up? A standard of care is the yardstick used to measure effectiveness of care.

Spotlight on NICE

The NICE is an independent organisation responsible for providing evidence-based national guidance on all aspects of healthcare.

NICE guidance is developed by a number of independent advisory groups made up of health professionals, those working in the NHS, patients, their carers and the public.

NICE produces guidance in three areas of health:

- public health – guidance on the promotion of good health and the prevention of ill-health for those working in the NHS, local authorities and the wider public and voluntary sector
- health technologies – guidance on the use of new and existing medicines, treatments and procedures within the NHS
- clinical practice – guidance on the appropriate treatment and care of people with specific diseases and conditions within the NHS.

Health Care Commission (HCC) and Health Care Standards Unit (HCSU)

The HCC is the independent watchdog for healthcare in the UK. The HCC is responsible for assessing and reporting on the services provided by all NHS and independent healthcare organisations. The HCC also actively promote improvements in standards of care and provide information on service performance to the public.

The HCSU works with the Department of Health to develop and maintain the Standards for better Health (SfBH). The standards are used in the assessment processes carried out by the HCC.

The SfBH are divided into seven domains:
* safety
* clinical and cost effectiveness
* governance
* patient focus
* accessible and responsive care
* care environment and amenities
* public health.

These general standards apply to all areas of healthcare and so must be considered when planning and delivering any healthcare service. For wound care specifically, they provide important guidance when establishing new services such as wound care or leg ulcer clinics or when auditing the standard of existing provision.

European Pressure Ulcer Advisory Panel

EPUAP was formed in 1996 to lead and support all European countries in efforts to prevent and treat pressure ulcers. Their mission statement is: '*to provide the relief of persons suffering from or at risk of pressure ulcers, in particular through research and the education of the public.*'

By going to the EPUAP website address (see page 275) you will find lots of useful information about pressure ulcers, notification of educational events and conferences and links to other wound-related websites and organisations.

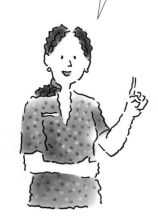

Nursing care specialists must live up to high standards established by specialty nursing organisations.

An ounce of prevention . . .

Clinical practice guidelines are systematically developed, evidence-based statements which aim to support clinical decisions in specific clinical circumstances. The EPUAP Guidelines for pressure ulcer prevention and treatment were produced in 1998 and 1999, respectively.
* 'Pressure Ulcer Prevention Guidelines' deal with tools to identify patients at risk of developing pressure ulcers, risk factors for ulceration, guidelines for external support surfaces and education.

- 'Pressure Ulcer Treatment Guidelines' include definition and classification of pressure ulcers, assessment of ulcer and patient, management of tissue loads and ulcer treatment.

In the decade since these Guidelines were published much has changed in pressure ulcer prevention and treatment and they are now in need of revision. In response to this, EPUAP are working with stakeholders in many countries including the US to produce International Pressure Ulcer Guidelines.

European Wound Management Association

EWMA was founded in 1991 to address clinical and scientific issues associated with wound healing represented by medical, nursing, scientific and pharmaceutical interests. The council was formed with members from the UK and mainland Europe. EWMA's stated aim is to: *'promote advancement of education and research into native epidemiology, pathology, diagnosis, prevention and management of wounds of all aetiologies.'*

Organisation and unit-specific policies and procedures

The policies and procedures in your employing organisation are also used to establish standards of care. Policies and procedures are commonly used in litigation claims. Too often, practitioners are informed of policies and procedures but don't take time to examine and understand them. Deviating from organisational policies and procedures can lead to suggestions of failure to meet the organisation's standards of care.

Job descriptions

Job descriptions play a role in determining standards of care as well. How does your employer define the healthcare team's role and relationships? Depending on the practice setting – such as hospital, home or extended care facility – your role may vary.

That's not in my job description!

To protect patients and staff members, firm practice guidelines are needed for all personnel to make sure that job descriptions are accurate. If healthcare employees practise outside their formal job descriptions, the employing organisation's legal advisors or insurance company could win a judgment against those employees to recover some of the losses incurred.

Patient rights

The Patients' Charter, produced in 1991, aimed to improve the quality of care received in the National Health Service (NHS) in the UK. It was abolished in 2000 under the 10-year NHS plan and the NHS now offers a more detailed list of Rights. These are grouped under the following headings:

- access to health services
- quality of care and environment
- nationally approved treatments, drugs and programmes
- respect, consent and confidentiality
- informed choice
- involvement in your healthcare and in the NHS
- complaint and redress.

These Rights form another recognised basis for standards of care. They apply to all aspects of healthcare provision and should be used to guide the delivery and audit of high quality wound care services specifically. The rights in full can be accessed on the NHS website at http://www.nhs.uk/Pages/homepage.aspx.

European Union Charter of Fundamental Rights

A further basis for standards of care is the European Union Charter of Fundamental Rights, as signed and proclaimed by the Presidents of the European Parliament, the Council and the Commission at the European Council meeting in Nice in 2000. The Charter encompasses the whole range of civil, political, economic and social rights of European citizens and all persons resident in the European Union (EU).

These rights are divided into six sections:

- dignity
- freedoms
- equality
- solidarity
- citizens' rights
- justice.

Unlike the NHS Rights, the European Union Rights are applicable to all aspects of life not just healthcare; however, they can (and should) still be used to guide the planning and delivery of any wound care service. It is also important for healthcare workers to know that any of these Rights may be raised as an issue by any patient who feels that one or more of their fundamental Rights has not been met.

The Rights can be accessed in full on the European Parliament's website at http://www.europarl.europa.eu/charter/default_en.htm

Litigation

Litigation is a lawsuit that's contested in court to enforce a right or pursue a resolution. Examples of legal liability specifically related to wound care usually involve claims of negligence, such as:

- failure to prevent
- failure to treat
- failure to heal.

Negligence, which is now recognised as a form of malpractice, is defined as failure to meet a standard of care – in other words, failure to do what another reasonably prudent healthcare provider would do in similar circumstances.

Malpractice is a healthcare professional's wrongful conduct, improper discharge of professional duties or failure to meet standards of care that result in harm to another person. Most malpractice litigation comes as a result of claims that a healthcare provider failed to:

- provide physical protection
- monitor or assess
- promptly respond
- properly administer a medication.

Practitioners in critical care, emergency, trauma and obstetrics and those who practise as specialists are particularly vulnerable.

ABCDs of medical malpractice

Four criteria must be verified to determine whether a medical malpractice claim is merited:

- A duty must be established with the patient. What this means is that the practitioner accepts **A**ccountability for the care and treatment of the patient.
- A **B**reach of duty or standard of care by the practitioner must be determined to evaluate if there has been an act of negligence or breach of duty that resulted in harm to the patient.
- Proximate **C**ause or causal connection must be established between the breach of duty or standard of care and the damages or injuries to the patient. In other words, the patient must prove that damages were due directly to the practitioner's negligence and that the damages were foreseeable. In other words, were the damages a direct result of the negligence?
- **D**amages or injuries to the patient must be presented as evidence as a result of the alleged negligence. These damages can be physical

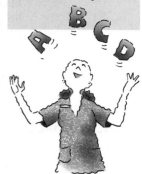

Memory jogger

To remember the four criteria that merit a medical malpractice claim, think **ABCD**:

Accountability rests with the practitioner.

Breach of duty leads to damages.

Causal connection is established between the breach and the damages.

Damages or injuries are presented as evidence of the breach of duty.

(disfigurement or pain and suffering), mental (mental anguish or financial (past, present or future medical expenses).

If the patient–plaintiff can establish these four components, malpractice litigation is merited.

Avoiding litigation

The key to reducing your risk of involvement in malpractice litigation is prevention. However, even if you provide optimum care to every patient, there's no guarantee that your actions will never be called into question in a litigation case. If that happens, you must be aware of how you're protected.

Practising independently without your own insurance is risky.

A common misconception

Many practitioners practice under the perception that they're protected by their facility's or employer's insurance policy. In most legal claims, your interests and the interests of your employer are comparable. However, the insurance company that provides your employer's coverage may be more allegiant to the employer than to you. In addition, the employer's insurance may not cover you if your performance fell outside your job description or if you didn't follow written policy and procedure.

The best defence

Excellent documentation is the key to minimising your liability because it's direct evidence of your evaluation and care related to wounds. The patient/medical record is your best protection and first line of defence. (See *Documentation do's and don'ts*, page 261.)

You must also be aware of your own limitations. Do not work outside of your job description or beyond your level of competency.

At your service

A patient's satisfaction with care also reduces liability. Typically, a malpractice claim represents the connection between patient injury and patient anger. Good communication with the patient and their family is essential to maintaining a good connection.

Healthcare is like a service industry, so you need to incorporate good customer service into your daily practice, including:
• Being respectful and courteous – people become angry when treated rudely.

Documentation do's and don'ts

To protect yourself against liability, document as accurately as possible by following these guidelines.

Do

- Chart factually, specifically and concisely – present your observations and interventions clearly and concisely.
- Chart thoroughly – malpractice claims are commonly filed years later and the passage of time impairs your ability to remember details.
- Date and time your entry – always make your entries as soon as possible after caring for the patient; delayed recording can lead to omissions.
- Sign your entry – if your signature is not easy to read then write your name in full next to it.
- Avoid making any changes or additions – if you have to change or add to the record ensure the original can still be read. Ensure you sign for making the changes or additions.

Don't

- Chart personal observations, opinions, feelings, or beliefs – these aspects of care are irrelevant.
- Use abbreviations, jargon or slang, or words or terms that the patient or client cannot easily understand.

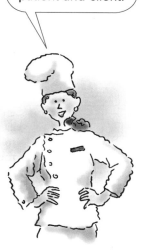

Make sure you dish up a healthy serving of respectful attention to every patient and client.

- Being attentive – give the patients the time that they need.
- Being sympathetic and empathetic – concern pays off in the long run.
- Being considerate and honest – patients recognise honesty, which makes them feel better about the care they receive.
- Recognising your limits – ask for help or a second opinion if you have doubts.
- Staying current – continuing education is a professional responsibility.

Record keeping strategies

NMC guidance on record keeping (NMC 2008b) states that record keeping is an integral part of nursing, midwifery and specialist community public health nursing practice. The NMC also state that record keeping is a tool of professional practice and one that should help the care process. Maintaining accurate and clear records helps to protect patients/clients by promoting:

- high standards of clinical care
- continuity of care between different carers and different care settings
- better communication and dissemination of information between members of the inter-professional healthcare team
- an accurate account of treatment, care planning and delivery
- the ability to identify risks and detect problems, such as changes in the patient/client's condition at an early stage
- the concept of confidentiality.

The NMC suggest that good record keeping is a mark of a skilled and safe practitioner, while careless or incomplete record keeping may highlight wider problems with that individual's practice. A good record should therefore include:

- an accurate and full account of the assessment
- an accurate account of the care planned and care delivered
- relevant information about the condition of the patient at any time; measures taken to respond to the patients/ clients needs
- a record of any continuing care arrangements
- evidence that the registrant has honoured their duty of care and that all reasonable steps have been taken to care for the patient/client and that any actions or omissions on the part of the registrant have not compromised their safety in any way.

In wound care, a structured wound assessment record (or tool) will provide a framework for thorough assessment and regular evaluation. Consistency of language and assessment criteria are enhanced, and improvement or deterioration in the wound is more easily observed. Risk assessment tools allow preventative measures to be put into place when required and provide an ongoing record of the patient's at risk status.

In a nutshell, good record keeping is imperative in healthcare, both for nurse and for patient. Well designed records (or documents) support good practice and allow audit pathways to be developed. Periodic training ensures staff members know how to use and complete documents accurately.

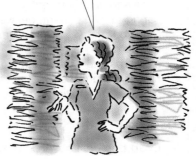

Documentation may seem overwhelming but it's incredibly important. Remember, litigation often stands or falls on the accuracy of the documentation.

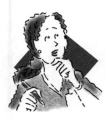

Quick quiz

1. According to The Code (NMC 2008) what should nurses make their first concern?
    A.   high standards of communication
    B.   the maintenance of up-to-date knowledge and skills
    C.   the accuracy of patient records
    D.   the care of people.

Answer: A. All these are important but The Code states specifically that nurses should 'make the care of people their first concern, treating them as individuals and respecting their dignity.'

2. Which European organisation developed the Clinical Practice Guidelines on the prevention and treatment of pressure ulcers?
    A.   European Wound Management Association
    B.   European Pressure Ulcer Advisory Panel
    C.   National Institute of Clinical Excellence
    D.   Health Care Commission.

Answer: B. The European Pressure Ulcer Advisory Panel produced guidelines for pressure ulcer prevention and treatment in 1998 and 1999 respectively. These are now under review.

3. Which describes an act of negligence that results in harm?
    A.   breach of duty
    B.   proximal cause
    C.   causal connection
    D.   established duty.

Answer: A. A breach of duty or standard of care must be determined to evaluate whether there has been an act of negligence.

4. The most effective way you can minimise your liability in a malpractice suit is by:
    A.   charting opinions rather than fact
    B.   being disrespectful and discourteous
    C.   charting accurately, clearly, concisely, promptly and thoroughly
    D.   being inattentive.

Answer: C. Accurately charting is your best protection to minimise your liability in a malpractice suit.

5. A good record should:
   A. show that duty of care has been honoured
   B. be written on a weekly basis
   C. be completed in pencil
   D. be completed by the most senior person on duty.

Answer: A. Show that duty of care has been honoured and that all reasonable steps have been taken to care for the patient/client and that any actions or omissions on the part of the registrant have not compromised their safety in any way.

Scoring

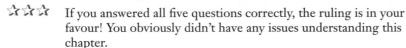

☆☆☆ If you answered all five questions correctly, the ruling is in your favour! You obviously didn't have any issues understanding this chapter.

☆☆ If you answered four questions correctly, don't judge yourself too harshly! But do brush up on the information you missed.

☆ If you answered fewer than four questions correctly, just call this a trial run! Prepare to defend yourself next time by reviewing the chapter.

References

NMC (2008a) *The Code – Standards of Conduct, Performance and Ethics for Nurses and Midwives*. London: NMC.

NMC (2008b) *Record Keeping – Advice Sheet*. London: NMC.

NMC (2009) About us. [on-line] [Accessed on 4th April 2009] Available: http://www.nmc-uk.org/aSection.aspx?SectionID=5

Appendices and index

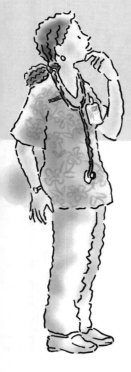

Pressure ulcer prevention algorithm

This algorithm forms part of the NICE guideline on pressure ulcer prevention. NICE have also produced a combined algorithm for both pressure ulcer prevention and management (CG29). Copies of all NICE guidelines can be obtained free of charge from the NICE website (www.nice.org.uk).

The algorithm should be read in conjunction with the full NICE guidance documents on pressure ulcer management and pressure ulcer prevention (CG29) and should be used to support clinical decisions rather than dictating them. Individual responsibility for making decisions appropriate to the circumstances of the individual patient, in consultation with the patient and/or carer, remains with the healthcare professional.

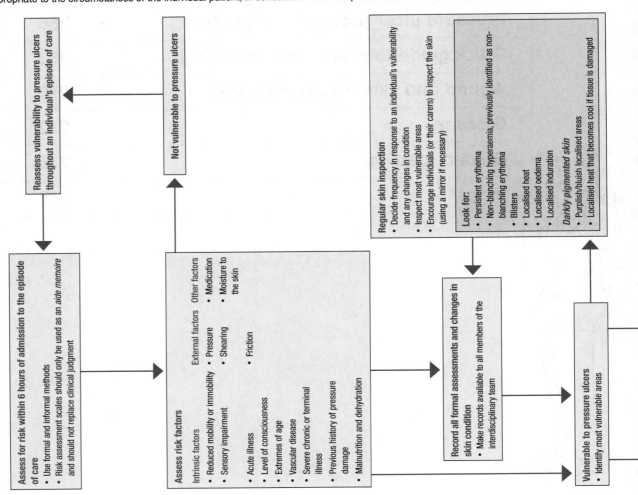

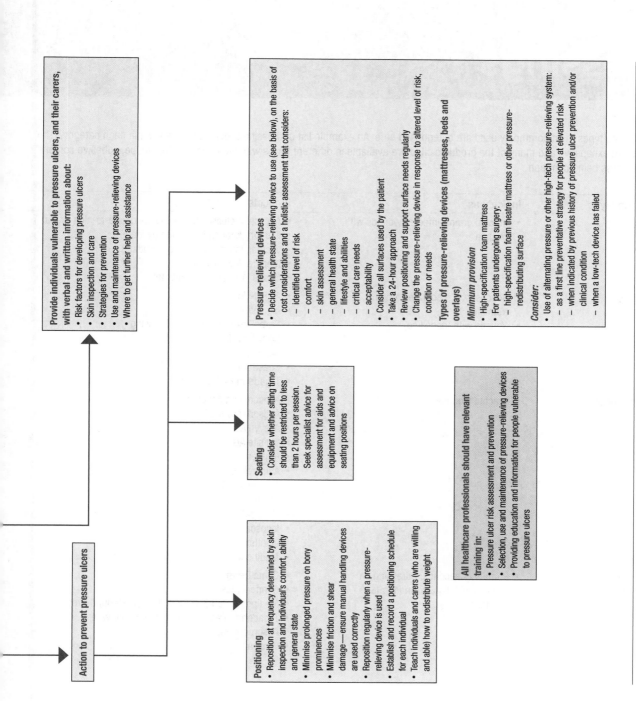

Action to prevent pressure ulcers

Provide individuals vulnerable to pressure ulcers, and their carers, with verbal and written information about:
- Risk factors for developing pressure ulcers
- Skin inspection and care
- Strategies for prevention
- Use and maintenance of pressure-relieving devices
- Where to get further help and assistance

Positioning
- Reposition at frequency determined by skin inspection and individual's comfort, ability and general state
- Minimise prolonged pressure on bony prominences
- Minimise friction and shear damage—ensure manual handling devices are used correctly
- Reposition regularly when a pressure-relieving device is used
- Establish and record a positioning schedule for each individual
- Teach individuals and carers (who are willing and able) how to redistribute weight

Seating
- Consider whether sitting time should be restricted to less than 2 hours per session. Seek specialist advice for assessment for aids and equipment and advice on seating positions

All healthcare professionals should have relevant training in:
- Pressure ulcer risk assessment and prevention
- Selection, use and maintenance of pressure-relieving devices
- Providing education and information for people vulnerable to pressure ulcers

Pressure-relieving devices
- Decide which pressure-relieving device to use (see below), on the basis of cost considerations and a holistic assessment that considers:
  - identified level of risk
  - comfort
  - skin assessment
  - general health state
  - lifestyle and abilities
  - critical care needs
  - acceptability
- Consider all surfaces used by the patient
- Take a 24-hour approach
- Review positioning and support surface needs regularly
- Change the pressure-relieving device in response to altered level of risk, condition or needs

Types of pressure-relieving devices (mattresses, beds and overlays)

Minimum provision
- High-specification foam mattress
- For patients undergoing surgery:
  - high-specification foam theatre mattress or other pressure-redistributing surface

Consider:
- Use of alternating pressure or other high-tech pressure-relieving system:
  - as a first line preventative strategy for people at elevated risk
  - when indicated by previous history of pressure ulcer prevention and/or clinical condition
  - when a low-tech device has failed

NICE (2003) *CG7 Pressure Relieving Devices. Clinical Practice Algorithm.* London. National Institute of Health and Clinical Excellence. Reproduced with permission.

Quick guide to wound care dressings

The dressing types most commonly used are categorised here. An example list of dressing products is given within each category. The lists are not exhaustive and many of the products cited are available in different forms with variations in size, shape, adhesive content and thickness being common.

Dressing type	Indications	Products
Absorptive	• Infected or non-infected wounds with exudate	• Aquacel Protease Modulating (moderate-to-high exudate) • Exu-Dry (moderate-to-high exudate) • Vacutex (moderate-to-high exudate) • Mepore (low exudate) • Opsite Post-op (low exudate)
Alginate	• Wounds with moderate-to-heavy drainage • Wounds with tunnelling	• Algisite M • Algosteril • CarboFlex Odour Control Dressing • Sorbalgon T • Sorbsan • SeasSorb • Tegaderm High Integrity
Antimicrobial	• Infected wounds	• Acticoat and Acticoat 7 • Actisorb silver 220 • Allevyn AG • Algisite AG • Arglaes • Aquacel AG • Atrauman AG • Biatain AG • Contreet • Iodosorb • Iodoflex • Medihoney
Composite	• Primary or secondary dressing on wounds with light-to-moderate drainage	• CombiDerm • Comfeel Plus • Medipore+Pad Soft Cloth Adhesive Wound Dressing • Tegaderm+Pad Transparent Dressing with Absorbent Pad • Versiva

Dressing type	Indications	Products
Contact layer	• Wounds with minimal-to-moderate; allows for flow of drainage to a secondary dressing while preventing the dressing from adhering to the wound	• Mepitel Silicone • N/A Ultra • Physiotulle • Profore Wound Contact Layer • Tegapore • Urgotulle
Film	• Partial-thickness wounds with minimal exudate	• Bioclusive • Mefilm • OpSite • Tegaderm
Foam	• Primary or secondary dressing on wounds with minimal-to-moderate drainage (including around tubes) when a low-adherent surface is important	• Allevyn and Allevyn Cavity • Biatain • Lyofoam • Lyofoam C Odour Control Dressing • Mepilex Silicone • PermaFoam • Tielle
Hydrocolloid	• Wounds with minimal-to-moderate drainage, including wounds with necrosis or slough • Secondary dressings (sheet dressings)	• Comfeel • DuoDerm • Granuflex • Hydrocoll • Tegasorb
Hydrogel	• Wounds with minimal or no drainage • Wounds with necrosis or slough	• Granugel • Hydrosorb • IntraSite and IntraSite conformable • Nu-Gel • Purilon • Tegagel

Wound and skin assessment tool

When performing a thorough wound and skin assessment, a pictorial demonstration is often helpful to identify the wound site(s). Using the wound and skin assessment tool here, the practitioner identified that the posterior of the patient's right elbow has a full-thickness pressure ulcer that's yellow in colour.

PATIENT'S NAME (LAST, MIDDLE, FIRST)	ID NUMBER	NAMED NURSE	CONSULTANT/GP
Stainer, Cathy	123-404113	K. Robertson	Dr. C. Payne

WOUND ASSESSMENT:

NUMBER	1	2	3	4	5	6
DATE	04/11/07					
TIME	0800					
LOCATION	R elbow					
SIZE-LENGTH	2 cm					
SIZE-WIDTH	1 cm					
SURFACE AREA	2 cm²					
TISSUE TYPE	SL					
WOUND BED COLOUR	Y					
EXUDATE	SR					
VOLUME	Mod					
ODOUR	MLD					
SURROUNDING SKIN	MAC					
P/U GRADE	111					

KEY

Grade:
- I. Non-blanchable erythema (Intact)
- II. Partial-thickness skin loss (abrasion/blister)
- III. Full-thickness skin loss (superficial ulcer)
- IV. Extensive tissue destruction inc. muscle and/or bone (deep ulcer)

Appearance:
- E = Eschar
- G = Granulation
- IN = Inflammation
- NEC = Necrotic
- PK = Pink
- SL = Slough
- TN = Tunneling

Colour of wound bed:
- RD = Red
- PNK = Pink
- Y = Yellow
- BLK = Black
- MX = Mixed (specify)

Exudate:
- 0 = None
- SR = Serous
- SS = Serosanguineous
- BL = Blood
- PR = Purulent

- UND = Undermining
- MX = Mixed tissue type (specify)

Volume:
- 0 = None
- SC = Scant
- MOD = Moderate
- LG = Large

Odour:
- 0 = None
- MLD = Mild
- FL = Foul

Surrounding skin:
- INF = Inflammation
- Dry = Dry
- MAC = Macerated
- NM = Normal

WOUND ANATOMICAL LOCATION:

(circle affected area)

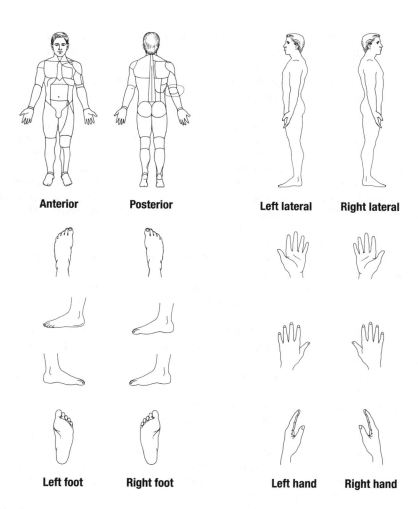

| Anterior | Posterior | | Left lateral | Right lateral |

| Left foot | Right foot | | Left hand | Right hand |

Wound care protocol: _Clean wound with normal saline_

Signature: _K. Robertson, RN_   Date _4/11/09_

Glossary

abrasion: a wearing away of the skin through some mechanical process, such as friction or trauma

abscess: a circumscribed collection of pus that forms in tissue as a result of acute or chronic localised infection and is associated with tissue destruction and, in many cases, swelling

acute wound: any wound that's new or progressing as expected

AIDS: acquired immune deficiency syndrome (AIDS) is a term that is used to describe the latter stages of HIV, when the immune system has stopped working and can't fight life-threatening illesses and infections

albumin: a large protein molecule that's water-soluble and provides colloid osmotic pressure

alginate: a non-woven, highly absorptive dressing that's manufactured from seaweed (kelp)

angiogenesis: the formation and regeneration of blood vessels

antimicrobial: an agent that kills microbes or inhibits their growth

autolysis: the breakdown of tissues or cells by the body's own mechanisms, such as enzymes or white blood cells

bacteria: one-celled microorganisms that break down dead tissue, have no true nucleus and reproduce by cell division

blanchable erythema: a reddened area of the skin that temporarily turns white or pale when pressure is applied with a fingertip

bottoming out: flattening of the support surface of the body, determined by the carer placing an outstretched hand (palm up) under the mattress overlay, below the part of the body at risk for ulcer formation (If the carer feels that the support material is less than 1-inch thick at this site, the patient has 'bottomed out')

burn: an acute wound that's caused by exposure to thermal extremes, caustic chemicals, electricity or radiation

cellulitis: cellular or connective tissue inflammation that's characterised by redness, swelling and tenderness

chancre: a painless (usually) ulceration fomed during the early stages of syphilis at the site of infection

chemical debridement: the topical application of biological enzymes to break down devitalised tissue

chronic wound: any wound that isn't healing in a timely fashion (healing has slowed or stopped)

collagen: the main supportive protein of skin, tendon, bone, cartilage and connective tissue

colloid osmotic pressure: the force that prevents fluid from leaking out of blood vessels into nearby tissues

colonised: contaminated with bacteria

contamination: the presence of bacteria, microorganisms or other foreign material in or on tissues (wounds with bacterial counts of 10(5) or fewer organisms per gram of tissue are usually considered contaminated; those with higher counts are generally considered infected)

cytotoxic agents: compounds that destroy both diseased and healthy cells, which should not be used to clean wounds; examples include Dakin's solution and hydrogen peroxide

dead space: an area of tissue destruction or loss that extends out from the main body of the wound, leaving a cavity or tract (this area is lightly packed to avoid superficial closure that can lead to abscess formation)

debridement: the removal of necrotic (dead) tissue to allow underlying healthy tissue to regenerate

debris: the remains of broken down or damaged cells or tissue

deep vein thrombosis: deep vein thrombosis (DVT) is a condition where a blood clot forms in a deep vein, usually in the lower leg

dehiscence: a partial or total separation of skin and tissue layers

demyelination: the destruction of a nerve's myelin sheath, which interferes with normal nerve conduction

dermis: the thick, inner layer of skin

de-roof: to remove the lid of a blister

diabetes mellitus: a metabolic disorder characterised by hyperglycaemia resulting from lack of insulin, lack of insulin effect or both

differentiation: the remodelling of collagen from a gel-like consistency to a mature scar (this maturation imparts mechanical strength to the tissue)

drainage: the fluid produced by a wound, which may contain serum, cellular debris, bacteria, leucocytes, pus or blood

eczema: an inflammatory skin disorder which causes dry, itchy skin typically in skin creases but can occur all over

embolism: a travelling blood clot that moves through your bloodstream and can partially or fully block lung circulation

enzyme: a protein that acts as a catalyst to induce chemical changes in other substances

epidermis: the outermost layer of the skin

epithelialisation: the regeneration of epidermis across the wound surface

erythema: an inflammatory redness of the skin caused by engorged capillaries

eschar: non-viable (dead) wound tissue that's characterised by a dry, leathery, black crust

evisceration: the abrupt protrusion of underlying visceral organs from a wound

excoriation: abrasions or scratches on the skin

exudate: any fluid that has been exuded from tissue or capillaries, usually due to injury or inflammation; it's characteristically high in protein and white blood cells

fascia: a band of white fibrous tissue that lies deep in relation to the skin and forms a supportive sheath for muscles and various body organs

fibrin: an insoluble protein, formed from fibrinogen by the proteolytic action of thrombin, that's essential in blood clotting

fibroblasts: the most common cells in connective tissue; responsible for making fibres and extracellular matrix, which provides support to cells

fistula: an abnormal passage between two organs or between an organ and the skin

foam: a sponge-like polymer dressing with some absorptive properties that may be adherent or impregnated or coated with other materials

friction: the act of rubbing one surface against another; may lead to the physiological wearing away of tissue

full-thickness wound: any wound that penetrates completely through the skin into underlying tissues; adipose tissue, muscle, tendon or bone may be exposed

gauze: a woven cotton or synthetic fabric dressing that's permeable to water, water vapour and oxygen and may be impregnated with petroleum, antiseptics or other agents. Not suitable as a wound contact material due to its tendency to adhere and cause tissue damage and pain

granulation: the formation of soft, pink, fleshy tissue during the healing process in a wound not healing by primary intention, consisting of new capillaries surrounded by fibrous collagen; tissue appears reddened from the rich blood supply

haemorrhage: bleeding (may be internal or external)

healing ridge: a build-up of collagen fibres that begins to form during the inflammatory phase of wound healing and peaks during the proliferation phase

HIV: the human immunodeficiency virus (HIV) is a virus that attacks the body's immune system

hydrocolloid: an adhesive, mouldable wafer dressing that's made of carbohydrates, has a non-permeable waterproof backing, and may have some absorptive properties

hydrogel: a water-based non-adherent dressing that has some absorptive qualities

hydrophilic: the ability to readily absorb moisture

hypovolaemia: a decrease in circulating blood volume (specifically plasma)

hypoxia: the reduction of oxygen in body tissues to below normal levels

induration: tissue firmness that may occur around a wound margin following blanchable erythema or chronic venous congestion

infection: a pathogenic contamination that's reacted against but can't be controlled by the body's immune system

inflammation: a localised protective response elicited by injury or destruction of tissue that's characterised by heat, redness, swelling pain and loss of function

insulin: a hormone secreted into the blood by the islets of Langerhans in the pancreas that promotes the storage of glucose, among other functions

irrigation: cleaning tissue and removing cell debris and drainage from an open wound by flushing it with a stream of liquid

ischaemia: deficient blood supply to a body organ or tissue

lymphoedema: the chronic swelling of a body part from accumulation of interstitial fluid secondary to obstruction of lymphatic vessels or lymph nodes

maceration: the softening of a solid as it's soaked in fluid (in wounds, maceration is indicated by whitened tissue)

macrophage: a highly phagocytic cell that's stimulated by inflammation

mechanical debridement: the removal of foreign material and devitalised or contaminated tissue from a wound by physical force rather than by chemical (enzymatic) or natural (autolytic) forces; examples include wet-to-dry dressings, pulsatile lavage and whirlpool therapy

melanin: a dark skin pigment that filters ultraviolet radiation and is produced and dispersed by specialised cells called melanocytes

myelin: a lipid-like substance that surrounds the axon of myelinated nerve fibres and permits normal neurological conduction

necrosis: cell or tissue death

neuron: a highly specialised conductor cell that receives and transmits electrochemical nerve impulses

neutrophil: a type of white blood cell that's responsible for phagocytosis

non-blanching erythema: a redness of the skin that persists when gentle pressure is applied to it and released

nutritional assessment: an assessment of the relationship between nutrients consumed and energy expended, especially when illness or surgery compromises a patient's intake or alters their metabolic requirements (includes a dietary history, physical assessment, anthropometric measurements and diagnostic tests)

osteitis: inflammation of the bone

partial-thickness wound: any wound that involves only the epidermal layer of the skin or extends through the epidermis and into — but not through — the dermis

pathogen: any microorganism capable of producing disease

peripheral vascular disease: a group of disorders that affect the blood vessels outside the heart or the lymphatic vessels

phagocyte: a cell that ingests microorganisms, other cells and foreign particles

phagocytosis: the engulfment of microorganisms, other cells and foreign particles by a phagocyte

polyneuropathy: damage to multiple types of nerves

potable: suitable for drinking

pressure: a force that's applied vertically or perpendicular to a surface

pressure gradient: the difference in pressure between two points (the transmission of pressure from one tissue to another causes an increase in pressure to those tissues that are deepest)

pressure ulcers: wounds that are the clinical manifestation of localised tissue death due to lack of blood flow in areas under pressure

prevalence: the total number of cases of a condition or disease e.g. pressure ulcers in a given population at a given time.

primary dressing: a dressing that's placed directly on the wound bed

protein: a large, complex molecule composed of amino acids, which are essential for tissue growth and repair

pus: a thick, yellowish fluid that's composed of albuminous substances, thin fluid, dead bacteria and leukocytes

pyoderma gangrenosum: pyoderma gangrenosum is a rapidly evolving skin disease typified by the presence of painful skin lesions/ulcerations.

radiation recall: a severe skin reaction that occurs when certain chemotherapy drugs are administered during or soon after radiation

reactive hyperaemia: an increased amount of blood in a body part following stoppage and subsequent restoration of the blood supply

sebaceous gland: a sac-like structure that produces sebum

sebum: a fatty substance that lubricates and softens the skin

sharp debridement: the removal of foreign material or devitalised (dead) tissue using a sharp instrument such as a scalpel

shearing force: a mechanical force that runs parallel, rather than perpendicular, to an area of skin (deep tissues feel the brunt of this force)

sinus tract: a channel-type extension of the wound bed into adjacent tissue; also known as a tunnel

skin sealant: a clear liquid that creates a film barrier to seal and protect the skin from trauma

slough: non-viable tissue that's loosely attached; characterised by string-like, moist, necrotic debris; and yellow, green or grey in colour

subcutaneous tissue: a layer of loose connective tissue below the epidermis and dermis that contains major blood vessels, lymph vessels and nerves; also known as the hypodermis

surgical wound: a healthy and uncomplicated break in the skin's continuity resulting from surgery

tattooing: permanent skin marking that can be caused by leaving embedded debris in a wound following traumatic injury e.g. asphalt

tendon: a fibrous cord of connective tissue that attaches the muscle to bone or cartilage and enables bones to move when skeletal muscles contract

tensile strength: the maximum force or pressure that can be applied to a wound without causing it to break apart

thrush: thrush is a common infection caused by a yeast, *Candida albicans*, which normally lives on the skin, in the mouth, gut or vagina; if the immune system becomes imbalanced the yeast proliferates

tissue: a large group of individual cells that perform a certain function

tissue biopsy: the use of a sharp instrument to obtain a sample of skin, muscle or bone for diagnostic purposes

transparent film: a clear, adherent, non-absorptive dressing that's permeable to oxygen and water vapour

traumatic wound: a sudden, unplanned injury to the skin that can range from minor to severe

tunnel: an extension of the wound bed into adjacent tissue; also known as a sinus tract

undermining: a tunnelling effect or pocket under the edges of a wound that's caused by the pressure gradient transmitted from the body surface to the bone

varicose veins: swollen veins, usually on the legs, that look lumpy and bluish

vascular wound: any chronic wound that stems from peripheral vascular disease in the venous, arterial or lymphatic system

vesicant: a substance that causes blistering

wound: any break in the skin

Guided reading

Bosworth-Bousfield, C. (Ed) (2001) *Burn Trauma. Management and Nursing Care.* 2nd edition. Oxford, Wiley Blackwell

Bryant, R.A. and Nix, D.P. (2007) *Acute and Chronic Wounds: Current Management Concepts.* 3rd edition. Oxford, Mosby

Dealey, C. (2005) *The Care of Wounds: A Guide for Nurses.* 3rd edition. Oxford, Wiley Blackwell

Dimond, B. (2005) Exploring the legal status of healthcare documentation in the UK. *British Journal of Nursing.* 14(9): 517–518

Edmonds, M.E. and Foster, A.V.M. (2000) *Managing the Diabetic Foot.* Oxford, Wiley Blackwell

European Wound Management Association *(2003) Position Document: Understanding Compression Therapy.* Available: *http://www.ewma.org/*

Hess, C.T. (2005) The Art of Skin and Wound Care Documentation. *Advances in Skin & Wound Care* 18(1): 43–53

McGreggor, A.D. and McGreggor, I.A. (2000) *Fundamental techniques of plastic surgery and their surgical applications.* Oxford, Churchill Livingstone

Ousey, K. (ed) (2005) *Pressure Area Care: Essential Skills for Nurses.* Oxford, Wiley Blackwell

Royal College of Nursing (2006) *The nursing management of patients with venous leg ulcers.* Available: *http://www.rcn.org.uk*

White, R. (ed) (2005) *Skin Care in Wound Management: Assessment, Prevention and Treatment.* Aberdeen. Wounds UK

Useful websites

Cochrane Reviews
http://www.cochrane.org.reviews

Department of Health
http://www.dh.gov.uk/en/index.htm

European Pressure Ulcer Advisory Panel
http://www.epuap.org/

European Tissue Repair Society
http://www.etrs.org/index.html

European Wound Management Association
http://www.ewma.org/

Judy Waterlow
http://www.judy-waterlow.co.uk/

National Health Service Clinical Knowledge Summary
http://www.cks.library.nhs.uk/home

Leg Ulcer Forum
http://www.legulcerforum.org/

National Institute of Health and Clinical Excellence
http://www.nice.org.uk

National Pressure Ulcer Advisory Panel (US)
http://www.npuap.org/

Nursing and Midwifery Council
http://www.nmc-uk.org

Surgical Materials Testing Laboratory
http://www.smtl.co.uk/

Tissue Viability Nurses Association
http://www.tvna.org/

Tissue Viability Society
http://www.tvs.org.uk/

Wound Healing Research Unit
http://www.whru.co.uk/

Wound Healing Society
http://www.woundheal.org/

World Union of Wound Healing Societies
http://www.wuwhs.org/

Index

t refers to a table; i refers to an illustration; **bold type** indicates colour pages.

t refers to a table; i refers to an illustration; **bold type** indicates colour pages.

t refers to a table; i refers to an illustration; **bold type** indicates colour pages.

t refers to a table; i refers to an illustration; **bold type** indicates colour pages.

t refers to a table; i refers to an illustration; **bold type** indicates colour pages.